# SEX, POWER, AND BOUNDARIES

BOOKS BY PETER RUTTER, M.D.

SEX IN THE FORBIDDEN ZONE:
When Men in Power—Therapists, Doctors, Clergy,
Teachers, and Others—Betray Women's Trust

SEX, POWER, AND BOUNDARIES:
Understanding and Preventing Sexual Harassment

# SEX,
# POWER,
## and
# BOUNDARIES

*Understanding and Preventing
Sexual Harassment*

## Peter Rutter, M.D.

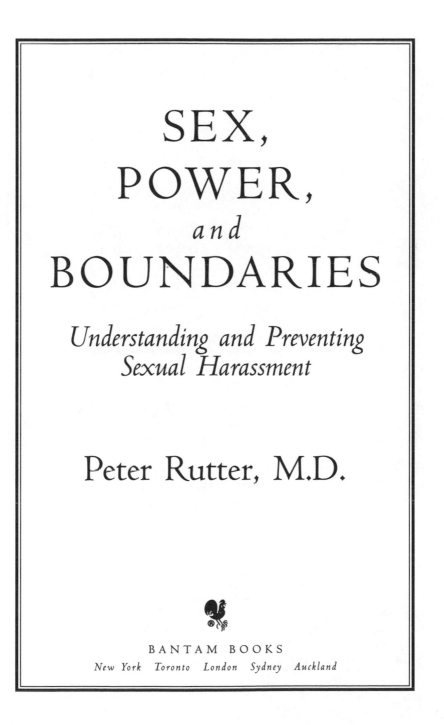

BANTAM BOOKS
*New York   Toronto   London   Sydney   Auckland*

SEX, POWER, AND BOUNDARIES

A Bantam Book / April 1996

Book design by Glen M. Edelstein.

Library of Congress Cataloging-in-Publication Data
Rutter, Peter.
Sex, power, and boundaries : understanding and preventing sexual harassment / Peter Rutter.
p.    cm.
Includes bibliographical references and index.
ISBN 0-553-09954-X
1. Sexual harassment—Prevention.    2. Sex differences (Psychology)    3. Sexual harassment—
Law and legislation—United States.    I. Title.
HF5549.5.S45R87    1996
613.6—dc20                                                                          95-47467
                                                                                          CIP

*Published simultaneously in the United States and Canada*

Bantam Books are published by Bantam Books, a division of Bantam Doubleday Dell Publishing
Group, Inc. Its trademark, consisting of the words "Bantam Books" and the portrayal of a
rooster, is Registered in U.S. Patent and Trademark Office and in other countries. Marca
Registrada. Bantam Books, 1540 Broadway, New York, New York 10036.

PRINTED IN THE UNITED STATES OF AMERICA

BVG      10  9  8  7  6  5  4  3  2  1

For Virginia Beane Rutter

# CONTENTS

# AUTHOR'S NOTE

I wish to acknowledge and thank all those who shared their personal stories of sexual harassment and enabled me to convey what sexual boundary tensions really feel like to both women and men. In the anecdotal content of this book I have protected the confidentiality of all individuals, other than those who are referenced in the Chapter Notes, by creating composite portrayals and disguising names, identifying details, conversations, incidents, locales, and the circumstances under which they provided such information. Similarly, except where specifically referenced in the notes, business and institutional names have been fictionalized, and any resemblance to actual organizations and companies is entirely coincidental.

In addition, under confidentiality agreements I consulted many professional colleagues with expertise in the field of sexual harassment, among them attorneys, academic researchers, government officials, psychotherapists, and human resource and other sexual harassment officers in workplaces and universities. I am deeply grateful to each of them for providing me with intimate access to these areas of ancient conflict and new opportunites.

There are also people whom I am able to thank by name for their resolute personal and professional support throughout my work on this book. I am deeply grateful for the collegiality and friendship of Fred Borcherdt, Margaret Clark, Pamela Cooper-White, Meinrad Craighead, Justine Beane Cunningham, Norman Cunningham, Joseph Henderson, James Levine, Suzanne Stricklin MacDonald, Nancy Novack, Ernest Pierucci, Andrew Samuels, Donald Sandner, Gary Schoener, Thomas Singer, John Steiner, Lynn Taber-Borcherdt, and Larry Taubman.

Richard Curiale and JoAnne Dellaverson, partners in life as well as in the employment law department of the McKenna & Cuneo law firm, deserve special thanks for allowing me to sit in on sexual harassment training workshops they so ably conduct, and for being available day and often night for discussions that always gave me new insights.

The Sociologists Against Sexual Harassment organization provided invaluable help from the moment I discovered its on-line Internet incarnation and at the annual SASH conferences, where state-of-the-art papers and round tables on sexual harassment are presented. I owe Phoebe Morgan Stambaugh, founder of the SASH-L Internet discussion list, special appreciation for her remarkable ability to integrate a sense of community with first-rate scholarship.

My friend and fellow author Paul Chutkow and my literary agents Maureen and Eric Lasher illuminated the path I needed to take and kept asking me, in the gentlest ways possible, to work ever harder at that alchemical task of transmuting intuition into words on paper. They are joined by Ann Harris, my editor at Bantam, who took scrupulous care that the manuscript might in the end live up to its promise. I thank you all.

Finally, my endless love and gratitude go again and always to my wife, Virginia Beane Rutter, to whom this book is dedicated, and to our children, Naftali and Melina, for letting me go to work on this book and, better, for being there when I returned.

# SEX, POWER, AND BOUNDARIES

# I. SEXUAL HARASSMENT

*Psychology, Law, and the Reasonable Woman and Reasonable Man*

At thirty-four, Steve Horner has made few mistakes in his rapid rise through the executive ranks at International Telcom. Already vice-president for national sales, Steve is highly respected for his hard work and innovative problem-solving, and he is a leading candidate for the company's future CEO. It is no wonder, then, that a huge knot forms in his gut when he arrives at work one Tuesday morning to find a memo on his desk asking him to come to an eleven A.M. meeting with Human Resources Director Betty Culverson, the company's chief sexual harassment officer. "Damn!" Steve says to himself as a wave of fear comes over him. "Sally must have said something to Culverson!"

Now thirty-one, Sally Dunheim has moved to the front rank of Telcom's sales force, spending half of her life during the last three years flying all over the country to help push Telcom's cellular phone service into the top five nationally. Sally tried hard to feel that it was an honor when Steve Horner came into her office after hours last Friday, congratulating her with a light kiss on the cheek upon her return from yet another successful sales trip. But an hour later Steve returned to her office, approached her, and said, "Sally, how about a *real* kiss this time?" Although she was able to blurt out a quick "No thanks," the incident upset her so much that after agonizing about it all

weekend, Sally decided to talk the matter over with Betty
Culverson the first thing Monday morning.

Sexual harassment cases like Steve Horner's and Sally Dunheim's don't
earn the headlines given to Professor Anita Hill and Justice Clarence
Thomas, to the U.S. Navy and the Tailhook scandal, to the jury verdict of
a $7.1 million award in the sexual harassment case against the Baker &
MacKenzie law firm, to the Senate Ethics Committee's vote to expel Senator Robert Packwood, or to harassment allegations against sitting presi-
dents or CEOs of major corporations. Nor are Steve and Sally themselves
avid followers of developments in civil rights law, psychological and sociological research, or federal court decisions that continue to define and
refine the meaning of sexual harassment.

Yet Steve Horner and Sally Dunheim, like millions of men and women
in workplaces and educational institutions, spend every day toiling
anxiously on the true front lines of today's sexual harassment problem—
where traditional ways of expressing sexuality now clash with federal law
and company harassment policies, where old rules, habits, and intuitions
about how you can or cannot look at, speak to, or touch a co-worker
fail us.

The headlines remind us all that the stakes are higher than ever—that
there are laws against harassment and that people are increasingly willing to
use them. But for most of us, the periodic major scandals and the historic
judicial opinions provide scant guidance through the thicket of everyday
perils. Today's workers usually register the reality of sexual harassment not
from newspaper headlines but from their own feelings and experiences. For
women, this registering often begins with the depressing knowledge that
the workplace exposes them to the same risk of unwelcome sexual behavior
that they are accustomed to elsewhere: behavior ranging from jokes, propositions, and comments about their body parts or sexual availability, to
being brushed against or otherwise touched against their wishes, and to the
far-from-impossible extremes of sexual assault and rape.

Accompanying this knowledge are women's fears of being labeled and
retaliated against if they resist or report harassment, along with long-term
feelings of resentment about being denied equal access to jobs and careers
because of sexual stereotyping. As Sally Dunheim exclaimed over the phone
to her friend Cindy the evening Steve Horner asked her for a "real" kiss:

You know Steve, my v-p for sales? I never thought he was coming on to me before. But tonight he comes into my office after everyone has left and gets real weird on me. He gives me such a strong sexual vibe, I'm afraid he's going to jump me. What *is* it with these guys that we can work together just fine for months on end, but at a moment's notice we're just *bodies* to them again? Am I overreacting? Do you think I'd be stupid to report this?

For men, the growing concern about sexual harassment engenders fears of doing something wrong—of losing a job, indeed an entire career, to a harassment accusation. Many men deeply resent the changes and lack of clarity in the rules of workplace behavior, and they wonder why they are now being penalized simply for behaving toward women the same way men have for centuries. Even those who try conscientiously not to sexualize their interactions with their female co-workers often live in dread that an innocent word, look, or touch will be mistaken for a sexual one.

In his meeting with Betty Culverson, Steve Horner—anxious, angry, and embarrassed when the sexual harassment officer asked him whether Sally had accurately described what had happened on the evening in question—blurted out:

Yes, I asked her for a kiss—she had already given me one, and she was acting like she was attracted to me. When she said no, I stopped, and believe me, I get the message. I'll never do it again. Is that sexual harassment? It was only as sexual as *she* wanted it to be! If she was offended, she could have just told me. Why is she coming to you about it and jeopardizing my career?

For men and women alike, the impact of sexual harassment law reaches beyond the workplace, invading homes by threatening jobs and economic well-being. It affects even our own intimate relationships by forcing us to question previously acceptable ways of flirting, dating, and declaring our sexual intentions; and it reaches deeply into our psychological selves, reminding us that the ways in which we express and receive sexuality can lead to experiences ranging from exquisitely loving relationships to a sense of utter worthlessness, terrible degradation, and irreparable injury.

Because the issue of harassment creates high tension about a matter as intimate as sexual behavior, in many workplaces bringing up the subject can create an atmosphere of uneasiness, silence, defensiveness, fear, anger, and even paranoia. Yet men and women long for reduced stress, greater clarity about how to succeed at their jobs and have good clean fun and friendly and relaxed personal relationships with co-workers.

Is there any hope that a sense of ease and safety can be restored to relationships between men and women in the workplace? A growing consensus identifies the more egregious forms of harassment, such as groping and crass sexual language, and labels them as unacceptable, but is there any room left over for innocent flirting and other nonoffensive behaviors with colleagues? Can guidelines be established that will allow men like Steve Horner to communicate their feelings to women without running the risk of offending them? Will women ever be able to count on going to work without fearing harassment or the retaliation that so often follows a complaint?

I believe that we can indeed find our way through the thicket of confusion about sexual harassment and discover ways of expressing sexuality that are healthy, respectful, and rewarding. What we require is a whole new body of knowledge and a whole new set of skills in understanding and managing sex, power, and boundaries—skills that our society, by naming sexual harassment and declaring it illegal, is now asking us to acquire.

The knowledge and skills I emphasize here have two interlocking dimensions: inner and outer. The inner dimension involves understanding the psychology and social conditioning that underlie sexual harassment; the critical role of sexual fantasy, especially for men; the definition of boundaries; the psychology of flirting and the dissimilar ways men and women send and receive sexual messages; the role of biology; and the identification of sexual and sex-role stereotypes.

Included in the outer dimension are the various types of boundary crossings and harassment, current sexual harassment law, company harassment policies, procedures for protesting harassment, and ways of safeguarding your rights, whether as someone who is harassed or who is accused of harassment. An important aspect of this dimension is the still-developing and often puzzling legal concept of the "hostile environment."

As we will discover, combining inner and outer knowledge leads to the most important harassment-preventing skill of all: recognizing and dealing with *unwelcome* sexual behavior. All sexual harassment law now centers on this concept. Because what is *unwelcome* can be misperceived, it is of central importance for both men and women to understand why misperceptions happen and to develop healthy boundary-management strategies. In the course of these pages, we'll find out what happened to Steve and Sally and hear about all sides of the harassment question, from harassers, victims of harassment, human resources officers, attorneys, judges, researchers, and therapists.

We will also discover that many disturbing questions and mysteries remain. Is anything about behavior between men and women fundamentally changed by the new emphasis on harassment? If it is, are the changes for the better or for the worse? Despite increasing clarity in the law and burgeoning company policies and training sessions, many studies show that about 90 percent of harassment episodes are never officially reported. What does this mean? Other research documents that the ten percent of workers, most of them women, who do report or file official complaints about harassment often suffer a negative emotional and job-related impact. Is it realistic to think this can be changed?

Larger social issues are also at stake in the area of harassment, including whether having to abide by new standards of sexual behavior in the workplace can alter the way people behave in their private lives. My view is that it can, and that at their most fundamental level the new standards point not to polarization between men and women but to a shared ethical vision of the dignity of the individual.

Because the roots of sexual harassment lie in the realm of ethics and values, I believe we have reason for hope in the changes that are under way. I have written this book with the same conviction that has guided my work over the years with my psychotherapy patients: that challenges, losses, even serious threats to our well-being offer us the opportunity to learn new skills and to meet stressful realities while preserving and even enhancing our health and integrity.

A major reason for my optimism is a pivotal development in the way our society thinks about sexual harassment. Early in 1991, two federal judges articulated what is termed the Reasonable Woman standard of harassment law, in the case of *Ellison v. Brady*. The Reasonable Woman standard recognized and validated the fact that women, because they have historically been disproportionate recipients of unwelcome sexual behavior, have a different perspective on sexual harassment from men.

The judges who established this standard, Robert R. Beezer and Alex Kozinski, had both been appointed to the bench by President Reagan. This is what Judge Beezer stated in his opinion:

> We adopt the perspective of the reasonable woman primarily because we believe that a sex-blind reasonable person standard tends to be male-biased and tends to systematically ignore the experiences of women. . . . We realize that there is a broad range of viewpoints among women as a group, but we believe that many women share common concerns which men do not necessarily share. For example, because women are disproportionately victims of rape and sexual assault, women have a stronger incentive to be concerned with sexual behavior. Women who are victims of mild forms of sexual harassment may understandably worry whether a harasser's conduct is merely a prelude to violent sexual assault. Men, who are rarely victims of sexual assault, may view sexual conduct in a vacuum without a full appreciation of the social setting or the underlying threat of violence that a woman may perceive.

When men allege harassment, Judge Beezer also wrote, "the appropriate . . . perspective would be that of a reasonable man." According the Reasonable Woman a place of equality next to the Reasonable Man suggests the possibility of true gender equality. It corrects an imperfection in the otherwise near-flawless perspective of the founders of American democracy in the Declaration of Independence:

> We hold these Truths to be self-evident, that all Men are created equal, that they are endowed by their Creator with certain unalienable Rights, that among those are Life, Liberty, and the Pursuit of Happiness.

For some of those who created the Declaration, the omission of women from this passage was innocent; at the time, the word *men* was widely assumed to encompass both sexes. But to other men of that era, this language was a clear affirmation that women were to be excluded from public life.

Yet it is from this original articulation of "unalienable Rights" that such values as racial and gender equality have sprung. In just under two hundred years, the pursuit of those rights has led to the abolition of slavery (1863); to women being granted the right to vote (1920); to the Supreme Court's decision in *Brown v. Board of Education* that racial segregation in public schools is illegal (1954); and to the Civil Rights Act of 1964, which protects people from discrimination of many sorts, establishes sexual harassment law, and lays the basis for the 1991 Reasonable Woman decision.

The installation of the Reasonable Woman alongside the Reasonable Man suggests that our society can now imagine new, more positive role models for men and women that make them equal partners. The bipartisan origin of the 1964 Civil Rights Act and development of the law since then are evidence that our society accepts sexual harassment law across a broad consensus, joining left and right, conservative and liberal, male and female. This consensus embraces the values of equality, common decency, and fairness for all. What follows in this book is dedicated to transforming the healing promise of these values into everyday realities for the increasingly reasonable women and men of our society.

# 2. SEX, POWER, AND BOUNDARIES

## *Mapping the Territory*

Before we explore the complexities of sexual harassment, it will be useful to lay out the psychological and legal territory involved, and to define some of the concepts fundamental to understanding and preventing such harassment:

- Sexual harassment as a legal concept, and its historical background
- Boundaries
- Sexual fantasies
- Flirting
- Feedback loops
- Notice
- Power abuse and gender harassment
- Sex-role spillover and reverse spillover
- Role modeling

### SEXUAL HARASSMENT IN ONE WORD: UNWELCOME

The behavior that we now refer to as sexual harassment is ancient. Throughout our existence as a species, some people have imposed their sexual words or actions upon others. Historically, women have been the overwhelmingly disproportionate recipients of such impositions, ranging from unwanted sexual speech, looks, and gestures to sexual assault and rape, and in a wide variety of settings, including the workplace.

Yet despite this endless history, the term *sexual harassment* itself is barely twenty years old. In her 1978 book *Sexual Shakedown*, Lin Farley describes how she and her colleagues coined the term for a course she taught in the fall of 1974 at Cornell University. The earliest media use that I have found appeared in a 1975 *New York Times* article by Enid Nemy, titled "Women Begin to Speak Out Against Sexual Harassment at Work."

Not until 1980 did a clear legal definition of the term emerge, and it remains the one in use in the U.S. today. In that year, Eleanor Holmes Norton, commissioner of the U.S. Equal Employment Opportunity Commission (EEOC) under President Carter, issued the following official guidelines defining sexual harassment:

> Unwelcome sexual advances, requests for sexual favors, and other verbal or physical conduct of a sexual nature constitute sexual harassment when (1) submission to such conduct is made either explicitly or implicitly a term or condition of an individual's employment; (2) submission to or rejection of such conduct by an individual is used as the basis for employment decisions affecting such [an] individual; or (3) such conduct has the purpose or effect of unreasonably interfering with an individual's work performance or creating an intimidating, hostile, or offensive working environment.*

Note that this legal definition begins with the word *unwelcome*. Following the definition come explications of the two different forms of sexual harassment: *quid pro quo* and *hostile environment*.

Sections (1) and (2) of the guidelines cover quid pro quo harassment. In this context, the Latin phrase (translated as "this for that") means that an employer or other person in a position of authority suggests to an em-

---

* In Canada, sexual harassment was defined by the Supreme Court of Canada (in *Janzen and Govereau v. Platy Enterprises,* 1989) as "unwelcome conduct of a sexual nature, which detrimentally affects the work environment, or leads to adverse job-related consequences for victims of harassment." It is illegal under Section 14 of the 1985 Canadian Human Rights Act. The European Community Code of Practice also bans sexual harassment, which it defines as "unwanted conduct of a sexual nature, or other conduct based on sex, affecting the dignity of women and men at work. This can include unwelcome physical, verbal, or non-verbal conduct."

ployee that he will give her *this* job, or promotion, or salary, in return for *that* sexual favor. Although quid pro quo harassment still occurs, it is universally considered so egregious that its illegality is no longer reputably challenged.

In fact, a male corporate attorney I know who conducts sexual harassment trainings often begins his presentation by briefly describing quid pro quo harassment, then looking out at the mostly male audience and remarking, "That's really all I have to say about quid pro quo harassment. I'm not going to insult anybody's intelligence by discussing it further. None of you would be here in this room today if you didn't already have the common sense to know how stupid and unacceptable it is. Now let's move on to the more subtle concept of hostile environment harassment."

This second form of sexual harassment is described in section (3) of the EEOC guidelines. Hostile environment harassment is the basis for nearly all the public debate, gray areas, and recent celebrated lawsuits and ethics charges. The unwelcome behavior involved can be classified in the following seven forms, listed in order of the frequency found in the U.S. Merit Systems Protection Board study, the most comprehensive government survey of sexual harassment:

1. Sexual teasing, jokes, remarks, or questions
2. Pressure for dates
3. Letters, telephone calls, or materials of a sexual nature (to which we can now add e-mail)
4. Sexual looks or gestures
5. Deliberate touching, leaning over, cornering, or pinching
6. Pressure for sexual favors
7. Actual or attempted rape or sexual assault

### The Evolution of Sexual Harassment Law: Celebrated Cases and Historical Landmarks

All the disputes concerning sexual harassment that have had a national impact in the past few years have involved a hostile environment, in which behaviors on the above list were alleged to have interfered with a woman's working conditions. Anita Hill's allegations against Clarence Thomas, which were raised during the hearings on his nomination to the U.S.

Supreme Court, centered around Thomas's having made sexualized remarks in alluding to pornographic movies he had seen, and in wondering aloud about someone having a pubic hair on his soft drink can.

In the Baker & MacKenzie case, in which the jury awarded legal secretary Rena Weeks $7.1 million, Ms. Weeks cited, among other behaviors, unwelcome touching from attorney Martin Greenstein when he placed M&M's in her blouse pocket—something that is difficult to accomplish without touching. The large award (which the judge later reduced to $3.5 million) was made not only for this behavior but for punitive damages, because the Baker & MacKenzie law firm, where Rena Weeks worked, was found by the jury to have knowingly tolerated past incidents of harassment on Greenstein's part.

In the Tailhook episode, Navy Lieutenant Paula Coughlin, together with several other women, stepped off an elevator at the Las Vegas Hilton and was immediately run through a gauntlet of drunken naval aviators, who aggressively fondled her breasts, buttocks, and genitals before she could escape. When she reported what had happened to the admiral on whose personal staff she worked, his response was, "That's what you've got to expect . . . with a bunch of drunk aviators."

Such incidents are considered hostile environment rather than quid pro quo harassment because, egregious though they may be, no one actually told these women they would lose their jobs if they did not participate in them. The message here is: You can stay on your job as long as you like, but if you're within target range of sexual behavior, you'll just have to put up with it. It is this message that enforcement of the 1980 EEOC prohibition against hostile environment harassment is meant to dispel.

It is important to understand the historical process that led to the EEOC guidelines in 1980. The pivotal event was the passage by Congress, with the support of nearly equal numbers of Republicans and Democrats, of the 1964 Civil Rights Act. Born of the civil rights movement for racial equality that gained strength in the late 1950s and early 1960s, and joined by activitists in the historic struggle for women's rights, Title VII of this 1964 act outlaws employment discrimination on the basis of "race, color, religion, sex, or national origin."

Although the act made employment discrimination on the basis of sex illegal, it was not until 1976 that a federal court, in the case of *Williams v. Saxbe*, ruled that sexual harassment is a form of illegal sex discrimination under Title VII. There are several other important landmarks in the history of sexual harassment law. In 1972 a Title IX amendment to the 1964 act banned sex discrimination, including what we now know as sexual harassment, in any educational institution that receives federal funds—which effectively included most American schools and universities. In 1986 the first sexual harassment case to be decided by the U.S. Supreme Court (*Meritor v. Vinson*) unanimously upheld the 1980 EEOC statement that a sexually hostile environment constitutes sexual harassment. Early in 1991 Judge Robert Beezer handed down the Reasonable Woman decision in *Ellison v. Brady*. (See Chapter I.) In October of that same year, the Anita Hill–Clarence Thomas dispute brought the subject of sexual harassment to the forefront of the national consciousness. And toward the end of 1991, Congress passed important legislation allowing for increased damages against employers in sexual harassment lawsuits. In 1993 the Supreme Court revisited the hostile environment concept and reaffirmed it in *Harris v. Forklift Systems*, adding that a harassee does not have to prove that she has been damaged psychologically by the harassment, but only that the behavior took place, that it was unwelcome, and that it would be offensive to a reasonable person.

### Preventing Nervous Breakdowns: Justice O'Connor Speaks Out in *Harris v. Forklift Systems*

For a woman bringing a harassment charge, not having to prove that she was psychologically damaged makes it easier to establish that harassment occurred and removes her psychological state from the central focus of the case, saving her from further invasions of privacy. As Justice Sandra Day O'Connor aptly and somewhat ironically put it in the Court's unanimous opinion, sexual harassment law "comes into play *before* the harassing conduct leads to a nervous breakdown" (emphasis mine). This was a case where, in Justice O'Connor's words,

> throughout [Teresa] Harris' time at Forklift, Hardy [her supervisor] often insulted her because of her gender and often made her the target of unwanted sexual innuendos. Hardy told Harris on several occasions, in the presence of other employees, "You're a woman, what do you know" and "We need a man as the rental

manager"; at least once he told her she was "a dumb ass woman."

Again, in front of others, he suggested that the two of them "go to the Holiday Inn to negotiate [Harris'] raise." Hardy occasionally asked Harris and other female employees to get coins from his front pants pocket. While Harris was arranging a deal with one of Forklift's customers, he asked her, again in front of other employees, "What did you do, promise the guy . . . some [sex] Saturday night?"

The Supreme Court's 1993 affirmation that Teresa Harris had been harassed demonstrates how rapidly the notion of hostile environment harassment is evolving. It came only after two lower federal courts had refused to uphold her harassment claim. In Justice O'Connor's words, the U.S. District Court that first heard the case found it "to be a 'close case,' but held that Hardy's conduct did not create an abusive [a word the court said it was using synonymously with hostile] environment."

It is also a significant marker of the growing consensus on hostile environment harassment that the Supreme Court decision in *Harris v. Forklift Systems* was unanimous, including the support of the conservative justices Antonin Scalia and Clarence Thomas.

## BOUNDARIES, FANTASIES, AND FLIRTING: WHAT DO WE DO WITH OUR SEXUALITY?

Obviously, wherever women and men work, learn, and play together, sexuality will be with them. At times it will be judiciously introduced, turn out to be of mutual interest, and lead two people to find themselves loving and intimate companions. At other times, unfortunately, the sexual possibilities between two people will rest strictly within the fantasy life of only one of them; and if that person acts on the fantasy, the object of his or her desire will feel offended and invaded, or even battered or stalked.

Under sexual harassment law, the kinds of sexual behavior that were previously taken for granted, including innocent flirting and complimenting another's looks, are no longer assumed to be acceptable. Our society has carved out a legal zone in which long-entrenched practices and rules of sexual behavior no longer apply—and an enormous zone it is. Harassment law covers virtually every workplace and educational setting in the country, placing these locales, in which most of us spend so much of our time and energy, outside the private sphere.

For obvious reasons, this new reality is often a source of confusion and perplexity; after all, human beings are sexual beings. Three key concepts are used throughout this book to help in understanding the ways sexuality can lead to sexual harassment problems. These are *boundaries, fantasies, and flirting.*

## Boundaries

Essentially, *boundaries* are lines of separation and demarcation. Just as a city or state has boundaries that define what lies within it and what lies outside it, people have personal boundaries. The basics of boundaries are easy to grasp intuitively: They are the sometimes-invisible, sometimes-visible lines that separate me from you, what's mine from what's yours, my space from your space. But boundaries also have subtle and complex aspects that can easily lead to misunderstandings because they mark out psychological as well as physical space.

The *sexual boundary* is the line each of us draws around ourselves in regard to sending out or receiving sexual behavior, whether verbal or nonverbal. Ideally, each of us should exercise control over our sexual boundaries. This means that we have the right not to be exposed to boundary-crossing—or even to *attempted* boundary-crossing, sexual behavior that we do not welcome. But maintaining our sexual boundaries also means that we take responsibility for controlling the sexual behavior we express toward others.

Developing boundary skills is of paramount importance. We must learn to perceive sexual boundaries in ourselves and others, and to understand how people communicate information about the kinds of sexual behavior they do and don't want. You cannot judge *unwelcome* sexual behavior, the prime ingredient of all sexual harassment, without recognizing how you yourself as well as the people around you perceive and manage their sexual boundaries. It is only *after* a sexual behavior, of whatever degree, has crossed someone's boundaries that the question arises of whether it was welcome or unwelcome. A great deal of sexual harassment can be prevented if we can make accurate judgments about what another person's reaction to our behavior will be.

Every actual or purported case of sexual harassment involves a serious disagreement about boundaries. The main categories of dispute are usually twofold: One is about how much space any person can rightfully declare to be within his or her personal boundaries; the other concerns the rules of boundary behavior in a specific workplace.

For example, Arianna walks down the hallway at work and notices a man who seems to be looking at her, as she terms it, "up and down." He's about twenty feet away. She ignores him and goes about her business, which she can do because she feels he is far enough away that her personal space is not invaded. But the next day the man stands five feet from her and does the same thing. This time she definitely feels that her boundaries have been crossed, that this man's behavior has been sexual in nature, and that it is certainly not welcome.

Let's assume Arianna complains about this second incident to Janet, her human resources officer. Janet has no difficulty concurring with Arianna that it was reasonable for her to have felt that unwelcome sexual behavior occurred. The boundary crossing is agreed upon. But the degree to which this behavior will be seen as sexually harassing depends on the second point of contention: What are the rules of boundary behavior in this workplace? Indeed, when Janet interviews the man in question about the incident, he doesn't deny the behavior but asks Janet, "Is there a rule against *looking* at someone?"

Before the articulation of sexual harassment law, certainly, there was no "rule against looking." Now there are some rules against looking (and against many other kinds of behavior) *if* the looking is determined to be unwelcome boundary-crossing behavior that to a reasonable person is sexual in nature and contributes to the creation of a hostile working environment.

As is clear from this one example and will be evident throughout these pages, boundaries and boundary crossings are complex matters but crucial to understanding and preventing sexual harassment.

### Fantasies

*Sexual fantasies* are scenarios of a sexual nature that we play and replay in our imaginations. While having fantasies is completely natural, it is critically important for us to manage our sexual fantasies in ways that do not lead us to impose them upon others.

Like all fantasies, sexual fantasies represent what is going on in our inner world. But the only way we can judge whether our sexual behavior is going to be welcomed by another person is to pick up cues from our outer, social world. The healthy management of sexual boundaries entails being aware of how completely different the world of fantasy is from the social world, and having the ability to relocate ourselves out of the fantasy world and into the social world whenever our sexual behavior may be affecting someone else.

Although this distinction between fantasy world and social world may seem obvious, an ongoing vulnerability of the human condition is that we easily become confused between our inner and outer worlds, especially in matters involving sexuality. Let's get back to Steve Horner and Sally Dunheim, whom we met in the first chapter. When Steve told his human resources director that Sally "was acting like she was attracted to me," he was fantasizing that attraction. His improper boundary behavior toward Sally was based on his fantasy, allowing it to justify asking her for a "real kiss."

For many of us, regardless of gender, the fantasy that someone is sexually attracted to us can be compelling. It certainly feels better to imagine so than to have to acknowledge that he or she may not be attracted. In other words, we are prone to prefer the message of the fantasy rather than absorb the less appealing reality. This is what happened to Steve, with the result that he subjected Sally to unwelcome sexual behavior. In Chapter 4 we will examine in detail the relationship between sexual fantasies and sexually harassing behavior, including the special vulnerability men have to putting their fantasies into action.

### Flirting

*Flirting* is a complex form of communication in which one person sends out encoded sexual messages to another person in an attempt to discover whether the recipient reciprocates the sexual interest. Ideally, two people flirt willingly and thereby come to a mutual understanding of how each sets the sexual boundary with the other.

But it is easy to see how things can go wrong with this form of communication. What if one person misreads the other's signals? Especially dangerous, and a common scenario in sexual harassment problems, is a situation in which one person has sent what she thinks is a "stop" message, but the other person reads it as a "go." After all, people flirt not only in order to pave the way for welcome sexual behavior, but to establish boundaries beyond which such behavior is not welcome.

Even more common is the situation in which only one person is doing the flirting, and the other person is not the slightest bit interested. In such a case, even mild flirting, if it persists, can be experienced as unwelcome sexual behavior.

Chapter 3 contains an extensive discussion of flirting and boundaries, with emphasis on the different ways that men and women experience flirting.

### How Sexual Harassment Law Has Changed the Rules

Before sexual harassment law, there was no way to separate the appropriateness of, say, flirting as practiced at a party or a bar, and flirting as practiced in the workplace. At that time, if it was appropriate in a singles bar for Steve to ask Sally for a "real kiss," he had no reason to change his behavior in the workplace. The common element—a woman who interested him— outweighed the difference in setting.

All that changed with the enactment of the EEOC guidelines in 1980. Sexual harassment law has imposed a major shift in what constitutes acceptable conduct in the workplace. Altering entrenched behaviors can be difficult; it requires learning new skills for dealing with fantasies, flirting, and other sexual expressions that impact on people's boundaries. Recognizing the lag between the time when average male expressions of sexuality went unquestioned by the society at large, and the present, when sexual harassment laws constrain such behavior, is one way of understanding what leads to many cases of sexual harassment.

In fact, one of the earliest sexual harassment cases to reach a federal court (*Corne v. Bausch & Lomb*, 1975) was unsuccessful for the woman who sued precisely because the judge accepted the normalcy of these male expressions of sexuality. The court rejected the woman's claim against her employer for sexual advances he had made to her at work as not being work-related and therefore not coming under the law—because, in the judge's words, "By his alleged sexual advances, [the defendant] was satisfying a personal urge."

This is not to say that before 1980 "satisfying personal urges" was necessarily the accepted standard of male sexual expression—or, as Lieutenant Coughlin's admiral put it, "what you've got to expect . . . with a bunch of drunk aviators." Male behavior, on its own and without the intervention of public policy, has always had its thoughtful, considerate, "reasonable" manifestations as well as its more offensive ones.

But because before the EEOC guidelines the views of women about boundary behavior were not legally coequal to the views of men, men have now been put in the position of having to learn that boundary standards that were acceptable in the past may not be acceptable in the present.

This does *not* mean that flirting and sexual behavior are now banned from the public sphere. Far from it. The new standard for judging sexual boundary behavior actually leaves ample room for conducting ourselves as we always have—but with one admittedly major caveat: those initial words in the 1980 guidelines: *"Unwelcome* sexual advances, requests for sexual favors, and other verbal or physical conduct of a sexual nature" (emphasis mine).

### New Rules, New Responsibilities

There is potentially room for sexual behavior under the guidelines, but the person who is initiating it has a responsibility that he or she has never had before.

This responsibility rests on the recognition that the workplace or educational setting has rules that differentiate it from ordinary (or even extraordinary!) social life. The baseline agreement is simply that we're here to work or to learn. Without this recognition, even the most innocent of workplace banter can cause a problem. Ted, a pension fund manager in his mid-thirties, was sent to me by his company for consultation (in lieu of a formal complaint) after Fay, a woman he supervised, told her human resources department that he would not stop commenting on the way she dressed. His remarks were always favorable, but she did not appreciate them and didn't know how to ask him to stop. Ted and I discussed his company's sexual harassment policy and the reasons why the woman might have taken offense.

At first Ted was resistant to altering his behavior. "I'm happily married," he said, "and I'm not sexually attracted to Fay. But I was brought up to believe that women like being complimented on their appearance. There's nothing sexual about that. I've been doing it all of my adult life, and don't see why I should have to stop now."

A few weeks later, Ted returned to say, "You know, I've been thinking about what I told you. I guess I have to concede that just because I was brought up in certain ways doesn't mean I get to make the rules about what's acceptable behavior. Women seem to be saying that they don't want to be treated at work as if they're in a social situation. I guess I can still compliment people all I want in my private life."

## FEEDBACK LOOPS AND NOTICE:
## JUDGING THE EXPERIENCE OF OTHERS

As Ted discovered, the new standard of what constitutes sexual harassment is not the motivation or intent of the person exhibiting the sexual behavior. Rather, boundary-testing behavior in the workplace is now judged by how welcome or unwelcome that behavior is to the *recipient*, as long as he or she is being reasonable about it. To prevent sexual harassment, each of us must understand that it is also our responsibility, whatever form the boundary testing takes, to make a judgment call about whether our behavior, sexualized or not, will or will not be welcome by the other person.

### Feedback Loops

Central to the skills of judging welcomeness are the concepts of *feedback loops* and *notice*. Feedback loops are fundamental to the art and science of human communication. We need them if we are to develop intelligent and well-balanced responses to the people and the world around us. The information we receive—the feedback—as a result of our behavior allows us to adjust our future behavior, forming a feedback loop. If we correctly perceive the relevant information being fed back to us, it will help us make accurate "reads" of others and adjust our behavior accordingly.

A great deal of sexual harassment prevention involves nothing more than using these reads to decide whether a given act on our part will (1) impact on someone else's sexual boundary and (2) be perceived as welcome. People who get in trouble with harassing behavior do not make effective use of feedback loops. Like Steve in his reading of Sally, they often use information from their sexual fantasies instead of information from feedback loops in judging sexual boundary situations.

### Notice

*Notice* is the process by which a person who receives unwelcome behavior makes it known that it is unwelcome. Giving notice and taking notice are also important parts of the legal equation in determining whether a given behavior is sexually harassing.

In harassment cases, the question of whether adequate notice of unwelcomeness has been communicated to the alleged harasser is often the core issue. Yet notice of unwelcomeness is more likely to be communicated indirectly and often nonverbally than in explicit verbal terms. When someone walks away from a water cooler where sexual jokes are being exchanged, it can be considered adequate notice that the jokes were unwelcome. At times notice is also served simply by the absence of any response at all. Because of the subtleties of how notice is communicated, we must all keep refining our feedback loop skills in order to recognize it.

For instance, Ted might conceivably be able to defend his repeated comments on Fay's appearance by proclaiming that he wasn't "sexually attracted to her." But if Fay finds his comments unwelcome and communicates this to him in some way, Ted is responsible thereafter for understanding that his statements are unwelcome. He has another responsibility as well: to develop the skill to refrain from making such comments in the future.

At first glance, recognizing and heeding notice might seem difficult: After all, how can I know the impact of my behavior on someone *before* I do it? Indeed, men who are being asked to learn new boundary behavior have an understandable grievance when they say, "It doesn't seem fair that I can get fired for doing something next month that was okay to do last month!"

There are several ways to meet this standard and recognize notice of unwelcomeness. First, it should be emphasized that it is very unusual for someone to be found guilty of sexual harassment because he did not know *in advance* that his behavior would not be welcomed. It is extremely rare for a formal charge to be made based upon one-time behavior; there is almost always a pattern of continuing boundary encroachments. It takes an egregious single act to sustain a harassment charge, such as touching someone's breasts or genital area, or shouting out sexual and aggressive content in an assaultive way. Behaviors like these would have to be perceived as being committed by someone who, by any reasonable judgment, has lost control of his physical or verbal boundaries.

Beyond these rare instances, recognizing notice of unwelcomeness depends on how well our feedback loops function. Equally important, the feedback loop for judging the effect of our boundary behavior has to be functioning at all times.

This vigilance can be difficult to maintain. Even proper notice of unwelcome behavior must compete with the many other things that men who are attracted to women in the workplace tend to "notice." As Sam, a man whose company disciplined him for sexual harassment, told me, "I can understand it if a woman just says to you right to your face that she's not interested in you. But the way they dress is telling us the opposite. What am I supposed to think, seeing them walk around showing their panty lines and the lingerie under their blouses? My brain can hear one message, but my hormones are getting a different one!"

Sam went on to admit, "To tell you the truth, at that point I wasn't even listening to what she was saying—I was completely wrapped up in how I felt." For many such men, the sexual fantasy that interferes with the recognition of perfectly adequate notice can frequently lead to sexual harassment.

Two women who consulted me, both involved in lawsuits, had very different takes on the question of notice. Beth had quit her job as a medical receptionist rather than directly confront one of the doctors about his constant brushings against her body. "Every single time he came near me," she said, "I walked in the other direction as diplomatically as I could. Either that wasn't notice enough for him or I need to work in a place with much wider corridors." But Tessa, whose boss had in his view "picked some lint off the front of her blouse" for three weeks running, was outraged that the opposing lawyer suggested she had given no notice because she had just stood there when these incidents occurred. "He walks by and feels me up," she said indignantly, "and it's my job to tell him he *can't?*"

## POWER ABUSE: GENDER HARASSMENT AND QUID PRO QUO

An important type of harassment, which is described more extensively in Chapter 5, is not really sexual at all. Called *gender harassment,* it is hateful, angry, aggressive, and demeaning behavior expressed toward someone on the basis of that person's gender. It is more like racism and other bigotries than a misplaced sense of sexual boundaries.

Rather than originating from a lack of clarity about other people's sexual boundaries, gender harassment as a rule is an attempt to exert power over someone, usually of the opposite sex, who is vulnerable and relatively powerless. Although power usually plays an important part in sexual harassment, in gender harassment the power is asserted directly, rather than through the filter of sexuality.

Women are by far the most frequent targets of gender harassment. Yet it can happen to men too. Al, a social worker at a small nonprofit agency, came to see me to work on some problems with his girlfriend. In the course of our work, his underlying anxiety emerged—he was afraid he'd lose his job. A conscientious man, he was the last male social worker left at the agency after the previous executive director, a man, resigned following a charge of harassment. The woman who had taken over as executive director had been curt and unfriendly to him from the start and was given to making comments around the office such as, "Men just can't be trusted to sit in the same room with women these days." She had also suggested that Al might have to be laid off due to budgetary constraints.

Because of traditional power hierarchies and the disproportionate number of men in the workplace, gender harassment usually targets women. But no person of either sex should either put out, or have to endure, gender-harassing statements of this sort.

Although quid pro quo (jobs-for-sex) harassment can be sexually motivated, it too goes beyond mere confusion about sexual boundaries. Because they explicitly threaten a worker's economic, career, and personal well-being, all quid pro quo incidents are abuses of power. Indeed, as a general rule in cases of sexual harassment, the more egregious the behavior, the more it involves power and the less it involves sex.

As has been noted earlier, "jobs-for-sex" harassment now accounts for a very small percentage of cases. This means that upward of 90 percent of sexual harassment cases involve an attempt to determine whether unwelcome behavior has created a sexually hostile environment. Thus, any attempt to figure out what behavior is welcome or unwelcome and to understand, define, and prevent a hostile environment must focus on the differences in the ways men and women behave at the sexual boundary.

## SEX-ROLE SPILLOVER AND REVERSE SPILLOVER

The pervasiveness of sexual harassment can be explained by seeing it as a subset of "normal" differences in the way men and women deal with sexual boundaries. Much of what is now known as sexual harassment may be a carryover into the workplace of the society's overall boundary habits.

The operative stereotype about boundaries is that men spend a great deal of energy pushing against women's boundaries, and that women in turn must devote a lot of their attention to figuring out how to manage men's boundary moves. The "normal" way of conducting ourselves in our social lives and communities tends to become the norm everywhere else, including school and work settings, where many boundary incursions are now legally unacceptable.

Social scientists have a term for behaving in public the way one does in private: *sex-role spillover*, a phrase first applied to the study of sexual harassment by pioneer researcher Barbara Gutek. It's a tidy phrase—it brings in *sex* and our learned, stereotypical gender *roles*, while the word *spillover* is certainly evocative of inappropriate usage and of crossing boundaries: We spill our familiar, stereotyped boundary habits over into school and the workplace. While there may be other possible sources of the sexual harassment problem, such as evolutionary biology and the expression of power in organizations (which researchers are now studying), in my opinion the commonsense notion of sex-role spillover contributes most to explaining harassment.

A particularly interesting, and hopeful, phenomenon is what I call *reverse spillover*. In reverse spillover, the new values of respecting sexual boundaries that are being articulated and enforced in the workplace are seeping back into people's private lives. Reverse spillover is the way the Reasonable Woman and Reasonable Man concepts make the transition from a citation in a federal court case to a living process that awakens people to a more developed sense of values.

### "Sure I Did It! What's Harassing About That?"

Sex-role spillover rests on characteristic disagreements between men and women about the very nature of boundaries and about how to judge boundary behavior. Increasing numbers of reasonable people of both genders agree in principle that sexual harassment, a hostile work environment, and unwelcome sexual behavior are bad things, but the definitions of almost every key word and concept having to do with sexual boundaries and harassment are virtually guaranteed to provoke a heated argument, with men and women in opposite camps.

Such an argument broke out dramatically at the first sexual harassment training seminar I observed, which was given by corporate defense attorneys for companies trying to prevent harassment. The male attorney who opened the day's proceedings asked the participants how they supposed a man was most likely to respond when first confronted by a supervisor about a possibly offensive way that he had spoken to or touched a woman co-worker.

Two women in the audience suggested that the man would probably first stonewall and deny the allegation. Then a male participant spoke up with the answer the attorney was seeking: that the man would likely admit to the behavior but minimize or deny its relevance to sexual harassment. The attorney affirmed that, in his experience, most men who are confronted with a harassment allegation for the first time will reply along the lines of: "Did I do that? Yeah, I did it! But sexual harassment? There was nothing *sexual* about that. And what's *harassing* about it?"

This response is often referred to by women, with an edge of sarcasm, as the You-just-don't-get-it-do-you? phenomenon, pushing the stereotype that men tend to be somewhat thickheaded creatures, unable to see what is perfectly clear to nearly all women. Yet most human resources officers I've spoken to report that when men are taken aside and privately alerted to the fact that someone was offended, more than 95 percent of them cease and desist engaging in the possibly offensive behavior.

## Human Resources and Other Role Modeling

Such reports of success with men who are "taken aside" buoy my optimistic assessment that most men are interested in being reasonable about sexual boundary matters. Assuming that women will also be reasonable, we could cheerfully assume that to solve the sexual harassment problem, we need only ask every potentially harassing man in the workplace to have a friendly chat with his local human resources officer. Absurd as this assumption might sound, it contains a modicum of truth.

According to the sex-role spillover theory, the harassment problem exists in large part because many perfectly decent (and reasonable) men have simply never had anyone tell them, clearly and credibly, that some of their behavior is sexually offensive to the women around them. Instead, role model after role model has taught each new generation of men that when a man has some sexual interest in a woman, it is all right to test her boundaries by exposing her to sexualized verbal or physical messages and seeing how she responds. But that was before the Civil Rights Act of 1964 and the 1980 EEOC guidelines came along to suggest that this generational tradition, at least in schools and the workplace, had to be reexamined and modified.

Denise, a graduate student in sociology, occasionally baby-sat for the children of Hank, her dissertation adviser, and his wife. She consulted me because the last few times Hank had driven her home, he had shut off the engine in front of the house and, in the cramped space of the car, tended to brush his hands against her shoulders and thighs as he engaged her in animated conversation about her research.

On the most recent occasion, he reached over and gave Denise a brief kiss as she began to get out of the car. She felt spooked, realized that her entire academic career was at stake if she alienated Hank, and was too shaken up to say anything. Now she wanted some guidance. I asked whether she would be comfortable if her department chair, a man named Richard, mediated the problem through a three-way meeting. Rather than confront Hank alone and risk subtle retaliation, a meeting like this might protect her interests by putting the issue on record with a third party.

Six months later, Denise happily reported that the situation had taken a turn for the better. She had asked for the three-way meeting despite her misgivings: Hank and Richard, the department chair, were good friends. She had recounted her experiences of unwelcome touch in their presence without directly accusing Hank of intentional misconduct. A few days later, Denise said, Hank had called her into his office, behaved like a gentleman, and apologized to her for his behavior. He told her that Richard had spoken to him in private thereafter, and Hank said he had been impressed and moved by Richard's ability, despite their friendship, to draw the line firmly and spell out why Hank's behavior was out of line. Denise counted herself lucky to have resolved the matter so easily. I agreed.

This kind of intervention is often more desirable than lawsuits and formal charges. But role modeling in which one man (like Richard) gives another (like Hank) a very clear message about appropriate sexual behavior goes against the grain of traditional male culture. Until recently there has been little public awareness of how important it is for men to hear from other men that their sexual boundary behavior has been offensive to women, and it is going to take time for such male-to-male role modeling to become more common.

## BUT ISN'T IT ALL BIOLOGICAL?

The way our society is redefining sexual boundaries affects men in particular ways. For them, the playing field has changed radically from an all-male domain to one in which women have equal legal status. Many men see this change as an intrusion on what they feel to be their basic nature. How, they ask, can society decide to regulate our sexual strategies and signaling patterns? Aren't these the most private, intimate, and biologically embedded parts of us? Millions of years of evolution are driving our sexual behavior, and now we're being asked to arrive at work tomorrow and stop coming on to each other? Give us a break!

"They can try to make us behave differently, but I really don't think it will work. My fantasies are working away all the time, and if a woman wants to cooperate with them, the fact that she's at work will never stop me." So said Joseph, an auto plant foreman, at a men's group in a sexual harassment training seminar.

When I went to an adjacent room to hear the few women at the seminar speak with one another, Lois, who had been working at the plant the longest, said, "Listen, girls, better get used to the sexual come-ons. First three months I was here, ten different guys came up behind me to 'help me out,' all rubbing me a little too closely. I ignored it—they were just testing me out. After I brought my old man around one day and they saw he's a big guy, it happens a lot less. But you can't stop 'em. It's just men, trying to mark their territory."

As Lois's and Joseph's remarks indicate, the resigned "That's just the way men are" attitude is still widespread. Some of this fatalism comes from long-entrenched cultural conditioning, and some from the assumption, like Joseph's, that biology drives the ways men and women behave sexually. Although no one can pinpoint the precise degree to which evolutionary biology shapes our social behavior, it obviously plays a powerful role. Nonetheless, our biologically evolved brains pride themselves on intelligent problem-solving in other, nonsexual areas. Even allowing for biological drives, I believe that it is within our capacity as men and women to respond creatively to the challenges of drawing new boundaries posed by sexual harassment laws, guided by the role models of the Reasonable Woman and the Reasonable Man.

# 3. SEXUAL BOUNDARIES

## Masculine and Feminine

There are basic differences in the ways men and women perceive and experience their own and each other's sexual boundaries: differences in how they flirt, strategize, and communicate; in how they guard their boundaries against unwelcome sexual behavior and attempt to negotiate welcome, intimate sexual boundary crossings.

Any discussion of these differences is bound to be heated, controversial, and marked by as many different points of view as there are people engaged in the discussion. Happily, such discussions are more open-ended these days than ever before. Older certainties that once constrained and stereotyped men and women are falling by the wayside. New ideas abound about what it means to be masculine or feminine, and more and more people are joining the dialogue, whether in worldwide Internet discussion groups, where anyone can register an opinion, or in select academic conferences that present the latest research supporting theories of either biological or cultural determinants.

The perspective of this book supports the continuing process of questioning, and at times redefining, what it means to be a man or a woman. To me, the most important goal of such redefining is to allow every man and woman to live unencumbered, as much as possible, by predetermined views of how he or she should behave. This means that whatever our statistics tell us about general patterns of sexual harassment, it is vital that each of us try to escape becoming a statistic. Just because high percentages of the people who sexually harass are men does not mean that a particular man is doomed to harass. Similarly, despite the studies showing that high percentages of women silently endure harassment rather than complain, we must encourage those who are harassed to step beyond those statistics, and we must make it safe for them to do so.

## MEN AND WOMEN: STEREOTYPES VS. DIFFERENCES

Because discussions of the nature of men and women often use the word *stereotype*, it is important to have a clear definition of the term. As used here, a stereotype is a fixed idea or image about a certain classification of people. Stereotypes—whether racial, religious, or sexual—are usually used in negative ways, to degrade whole classes of people or to devalue any one person by treating him or her as a member of a class rather than as an individual.

For that reason we need to move beyond stereotypes. Even when we do this, however, we are still confronted with certain patterns and statistical data showing that men and women are different. Because such differences can lead to problems, particularly in sexual boundary behavior, it is useful to look at five different, widely held ideas about fundamental differences between men and women.

1. Men are more action-oriented and thick-skinned.
   Women are more feeling-oriented and sensitive.
2. Men are more competitive and oriented toward creating clear chains of hierarchical authority.
   Women are more cooperative and oriented toward a nonauthoritarian sense of community.
3. Men are linear and logical thinkers.
   Women are nonlinear thinkers, and for them logic is secondary to emotion.
4. Men are providers; the workplace is their domain.
   Women are nurturers; the home and family are their domain.
5. Men are sexually adventurous and prefer sex with many partners.
   Women prefer monogamy and the security of a single partner.

What I say about these statements is intended to reduce negative stereotyping, while at the same time allowing us to incorporate the reality of differences that do indeed exist. I hope that readers will critically evaluate each of them and come up with their own opinions—opinions that may well shift over time. Ideally, these various assessments should provide readers with an opportunity for spirited and open-minded discussion, and even protests and disagreements with me.*

I believe that we have constructed a world in which all of the above statements are true. I also believe that many of these truths are lamentable—and potentially changeable.

On the other hand, if you add the phrase *by nature* to each of the five statements, I would disagree with all of them. We simply do not know enough to conclude that the differences that we have arrived at through cultural conditioning and stereotyping are the same ones that exist "by nature."

That is not to say that there are not differences of nature between men and women. Along with the visible anatomical disparities that serve reproduction are the underlying hormonal dissimilarities that make the anatomy work. Women in their reproductive years have a monthly menstrual cycle that differentiates their physiological functioning from men's, and biology has given them the capacity of conceiving, gestating, giving birth to, and nourishing their children from their own bodies. But the hormones produced by the endocrine system are not confined to reproduction; they also have multiple effects on the brain and on behavior. Because of this, it is possible that women have a better-developed talent for picking up on subtle cues about the relational needs of others. The research of Carol Gilligan and Deborah Tannen describes with great sophistication the ways in which women work to harmonize relationships around them, and how this is expressed through relational and linguistic styles that are more open-ended than those of men, in order to monitor for the feeling states of others.

This feminine relational style also affects workplace sexual harassment issues, in that women tend to monitor boundaries for different concerns from men. In general, a man monitors boundary behavior with more attention to cues about whether a woman is sexually interested in him, and has an added tendency to project sexuality into an interaction with a woman

---

* These can be communicated to me via the World Wide Web Sexual Harassment Resources site that has been established in connection with this book: http://www.bdd.com/rutter. They can also be sent directly to my e-mail address: pr@itsa.ucsf.edu

even when she has no such interest. In general, a woman monitors boundaries with concern for harmonizing relationships; she is less likely to look for a specifically sexual connection. In a variety of ways, such differences in boundary concerns can lead to sexual harassment problems.

Recent research on sexual fantasies—another major concern in harassment—also supports significant differences between men and women. Men's fantasies tend to be directed toward imagining particular sexual acts, the findings show, while women's fantasies, even when they are sexual, focus more on the emotional responses between themselves and the imagined partner.

Yet even granting that these variations exist, and despite what we think we can surmise from the gender differences in hormonal systems and reproductive physiology, none of these factors is sufficient to validate rigid notions of men's and women's behavior. Nothing about these differences has prevented women from serving on the Supreme Court, being CEOs of major corporations, or flying combat jets. Nothing has prevented numbers of men from being superb providers of love and nurture to their children, or from becoming deeply sensitive to the feelings of the people around them.

Some psychological theories, and visible evidence, support the potential of individuals to behave in ways that do not conform to the sex roles our society now presumes must prevail. As a Jungian analyst, I draw upon the theory of C. G. Jung, a Swiss psychiatrist who, along with Sigmund Freud, was one of the pioneers in the field of psychoanalysis in the early twentieth century. Jung felt that women, although encouraged to develop in ways that the culture considers feminine, also have the psychological potential to develop capacities that the culture considers masculine. His name for the so-called "masculine" potential of women was the *animus*. Likewise, he believed that men have the potential to develop capacities that the culture considers feminine. These culturally "feminine" qualities in men he called the *anima*. The feminine figures that appear in men's dreams and sexual fantasies, he felt, are actually inner images of that anima. This is a very useful model, as we shall see in Chapter 4, for men who are trying to draw back from their adaptation toward acting out sexual fantasies.

Jung's concern was that each of us develops our individual self as fully as possible, unimpeded by notions we have absorbed from our families or from our culture of what men and women "should" be like. In this respect, his is a hopeful and open-ended model for transcending sexual stereotypes that limit and degrade, and for moving toward gender equality.

One further biological difference remains centrally important to our study of sexual harassment—the simple fact that men on the whole tend to be larger than women. This means that, if they choose to, men can use force to impose themselves sexually upon women in isolated, one-to-one situations. Yet most men, even when possessed of this capacity, do not and never will impose themselves on women through force or physical intimidation, meaning that the differences between those who do and who don't use force is largely a matter of learned behavior, not of biological programming.

Therefore, although I agree that men tend to "push against sexual boundaries" more than women do, I take these tendencies to be a circumstance of the world in which we live today, not as an inalterable fact of nature. In my judgment, men possess these tendencies only because our society has historically given them permission to exercise coercion, intimidation, and even force in their sexual dealings with women. Although a so-called "locker-room" male culture continues to admire men for this kind of sexual aggression, our society is delivering more and more messages denying them permission to use sexual coercion of any kind. The clear articulation of sexual harassment law over the last thirty years is one of the most visible—and effective—ways of delivering these messages. These laws are forcing us all to be more conscious, and more humane, about how we use sexuality.

## MEN, WOMEN, AND BOUNDARIES

As defined in the previous chapter, boundaries are lines that separate me from you, what's mine from what's yours, my space from your space. *Boundary crossings* are any of the many things we can do, or try to do, to penetrate or cross the boundary between ourselves and others. We can cross the boundary with someone by speaking to them; by touching them; by looking at them; by sending them messages by phone, mail, fax, e-mail, voice mail, package delivery, or hand delivery; and even by anonymous postings in public places such as bulletin boards or bathroom stalls. We can even cross the boundary by throwing things at someone.

Every conceivable method of boundary crossing, or way of delivering something of *me* to *you*, has been at issue in sexual harassment legal cases, as well as in less formal complaints. Incidents of rubbing up against people, careless hands, and unwelcome comments have already been described. Written messages created the problem in the sexual harassment case that led to the famous Reasonable Woman decision in *Ellison v. Brady*. In this case, a male co-worker of Kerry Ellison's at the Internal Revenue Service wrote her a series of notes indicating he felt that they had a special relationship, although she had never indicated any such interest in him. The first note said, "I cried over you last night and I'm totally drained today. I have never been in such constant term oil [sic]." Although Ellison showed the note to her supervisor and told the writer of the note through an intermediary that she had no interest in him, shortly thereafter she received another one, saying, among other things:

> I know you are worth knowing with or without sex. . . . I have enjoyed you so much over these past few months. Watching you. Experiencing you from O so far away. Admiring your style and elan. . . . Don't you think it odd that two people who have never even talked together, alone, are striking off such intense sparks. . . . I will [write] another letter in the near future.

We will return to this note in the next chapter as an illustration of the fantasies that can lie behind boundary-violating sexual behavior. But to summarize: Name any method of boundary crossing, and someone has used it to behave in an unwelcome and offensive manner to someone else.

## BOUNDARIES AND SEXUAL BOUNDARIES

The *sexual* boundary, as it was defined in Chapter 2, is the line each of us draws around ourselves in terms of sending out or receiving sexual behavior, whether verbal or otherwise. This definition covers a great deal of territory, as it must in order to take into account the extremely broad spectrum of experiences and interpretations of what is sexual. Although much debate will be necessary to clarify different people's versions of what is sexual, we must begin by including anything that any individual *thinks* is sexual.

Obviously, how one defines the sexual boundary is fundamental to problems involving sexual harassment. My definition clearly includes those situations in which the two people involved, particularly a man and woman, disagree over whether anything sexual is going on. This kind of disagreement is at issue in many potential or actual harassment situations. Many workplaces, for example, have a notorious neck-rubber who thinks it is a perfectly routine matter to give people uninvited massages. So when Ed, the self-appointed office masseur, comes up behind Winnie and gives her a neck rub, he may think it is not sexual, while Winnie may think it is. Men also commonly joke about harassment. When a man jokes about getting harassment training so that he knows "what not to do," he may think that his "joke" is not sexual. Yet a woman to whom he tells the "joke" may reasonably experience it as a double-edged sexual innuendo.

Yet as inclusive as my definition of sexual boundary behavior may be, it does have an important limit. In saying that it is behavior that an individual perceives as being sexual, I intentionally exclude those situations in which something sexual is going on in one person's mind yet is absolutely unavailable to the other person. We are completely entitled to our fantasy lives and inner worlds. Fantasies, whether sexual or otherwise, need not cross another person's boundaries.

In fact, this is where most of the hard work must be done in order to bring about a society with new and healthier sexual boundaries—at the dividing line between what is within us and what is outside, between our thoughts and our actions. This is tricky territory because of the many ways that people tend to let their inner sexual thoughts and feelings spill over to others, sometimes without realizing it. A casual conversation around the water cooler can suddenly turn sexual from the perspective of either the speaker or the listener. Take the woman who couldn't resist saying loudly to nobody in particular but to everyone, on a very hot day, "I can't wait to get home and strip everything off!" A perfectly spontaneous and perhaps entirely chaste thing to say, don't you think? Nobody bothered her about it, but her comment did wonders for the fantasy life of the half-dozen men within earshot.

After Sharon Stone's famous police interview scene in the film *Basic Instinct,* I was told, water-cooler banter among men at a certain government agency included their taking bets about which woman that day would be most likely not to have underwear on. They did not always check to make sure no women were in hearing range; in fact, I was told this story by a man who himself found that talk embarrassing and offensive.

The truth is, nearly all of our efforts to prevent sexual harassment could be boiled down to this question: How good is your ability to keep your sexual thoughts and feelings completely inside, except for situations in which you *know* that divulging some of that sexuality is appropriate and welcome?

## SEXUAL BOUNDARY EVENTS

Many of the incidents already described in these pages are *sexual boundary events*. A sexual boundary event is any incident between two people in which either one of them feels that how his or her sexual boundary is being treated is at issue. When you ask someone for a date, it is a sexual boundary event. When you joke about sex in someone's presence, it is a sexual boundary event. When you whistle at or make eyes at a woman in a certain way, it is a sexual boundary event.

There are, of course, thousands of other examples, and we keep inventing new ones all the time. This does *not* mean that all such events are sexually harassing acts—far from it. Sexual boundary events make up a large proportion of the moment-to-moment life of the human species. Barbara, a computer programmer, was enthralled when her co-worker Nate asked her to lunch, then dinner, then for a long walk in the woods. These were clearly major sexual boundary events, but Nate and Barbara took them slowly, were aware of possible office tensions once they became intimate, and consulted the company's human resources officer for help on how to handle this issue. A more conscious approach to boundary issues can actually lead to happy endings—and theirs was one; they were able to keep both their jobs and their relationship. We will look in more detail at what is and isn't likely to bring about a happy ending in Chapter 5.

The point is that in order to make any progress in evaluating the welcomeness or unwelcomeness of a sexual boundary event, we must first establish that a sexual boundary event is occurring; then we can consider what its effect may be with greater awareness.

These events can be broken down into component parts, or stages, which I describe as *boundary monitoring, boundary testing,* and *boundary respecting.* There are important differences in the characteristic male and female approaches to each of these stages.

The differences show themselves at the very first stage. Boundary monitoring is the attention we give to tracking the messages we are sending out to others and those that they are sending back to us. As has been noted, there seems little doubt that men monitor boundaries for their sexual possibilities more than do women. Gary, an unmarried man of twenty-eight who works for a phone company, summed up a fairly prevalent male attitude when he told me:

> It's not as if I'm interested in sexual opportunities every time I relate to a woman; it's more like I'm always checking to see if I *might* be interested, or whether she seems attracted to me.
>
> But once things get to the level of my being interested, you can bet that, even though I try to stay cool as if nothing different is happening, from then on, no matter what's going on, I'm always checking every detail of her behavior for what it signals to me sexually. And even though I can talk to her in a way that doesn't *seem* sexual, I look for any sign that she is taking it sexually, because if she wants it to be sexual, then it is.
>
> Even if it's someone at work, and I say, "Lisa, would you like to check me out on this report I wrote?" I'll be checking out everything: the way she moves her body, her facial expressions, what she says, her *energy* toward me. It could be months, or never, before I'd do anything about it. But it's good to know whether something might be possible someday. You're not going to tell me this is harassment, are you? All the guys do this.

What Gary has identified is a pervasive masculine style of constantly *monitoring* the boundary for sexual possibilities. Stereotypical though it may seem, there is a wide consensus today that men tend to see sexual boundary events with comparative strangers as interesting opportunities, whereas women are more likely to perceive them as threatening and burdensome. Because of this, men can often say in all honesty, "What's sexual about that?" about everything from hanging around a woman's desk talking to her more than usual, to jokes and even to neck rubs.

## Masculine Boundary Monitoring: Levels A and B

Gary describes himself as always being aware of two different levels in his interactions with women. What we'll call Level A, the overt level of communication, can range from the businesslike to the gracious or downright disarming. But running simultaneously with Level A, encoded as if it were a second program using closed captions, is Level B, the continual internal sexual monitoring, the locus of a man's fantasy life. When Gary says at Level A, "Lisa, will you check me out on this report?" at Level B he's saying, "And if you like what you see when you check, maybe we can make something happen after work."

What men are really saying when they deny the sexual significance of their interactions with women is, "That wasn't sexual—that was just *normal*. If you want sexual, I'll *give* you sexual!" It's as if a man was insulted because you thought he didn't know the difference between Level A and Level B.

This division between Level A and Level B is not as crude as it sounds. The fact that men monitor so many of their interactions with women as potential sexual boundary events is not in itself a problem. Just because Gary thinks "Maybe we can make something happen after work" doesn't mean that he will ever broach Level B with Lisa. It doesn't even mean that he is secretly seeing her as a sexual object. It is important to grant men, and women as well, the full range of their fantasy lives.

As long as a man can keep his Level B information away from a woman, he is preventing a boundary event from becoming a *sexual* boundary event. The fact that, from the point of view of his fantasy, their interaction could turn into a sexual boundary event at any point should not be held against him.

Several years ago I consulted with a man named Rafe who, every week for six months, came to his meetings with me terrified that he had let his very intense ongoing sexual fantasies about Margaret, his supervisor at work, leak out in the women's health clinic where he was the office manager. Margaret had even asked him out to lunch and begun confiding in him about breaking up with her boyfriend. He felt particularly at risk because of where he worked, although with the exception of Margaret he had never had any boundary or fantasy problems with women co-workers or patients. Yet though he was careful not to reveal anything to Margaret verbally, he feared that if he walked too close to her, she would actually feel the sexual heat from his body or notice an erection in his trousers, in which case his career would be doomed. Rafe worked extremely hard with me on his fantasies, and his "crush" dissipated over the months. He is now CEO of a major national health care corporation, with a stable and happy marriage. And Margaret, who helped launch his successful career by giving him a rave recommendation for his next job, never knew about his struggle.

Ironically, the man who is insulted because of "If you want sexual, I'll *give* you sexual!" may actually be at lower risk to harass or otherwise cause offense at the sexual boundary than a man who isn't as clear on the difference between Level A and Level B. Kit, a man I once counseled unsuccessfully for telling more than one woman co-worker, "I like the way you fill a sweater," said, "It's all a sexual game out there, anyway. I'm not going to lie about what I'm putting out. The way I was raised, if a woman tells me no, I'll stop, but I have no problem letting her know I'm interested." I don't know where Kit is working now, but it isn't for the firm that sent him to see me.

Nonetheless, for many men it is a matter of honor to recognize the difference between the two levels and to decide for themselves which level they are operating on. Although it takes more than this particular distinction to avoid sexually offensive behavior, men who perceive the difference are light-years ahead of those who do not. Gary knows that he can operate at Levels A and B at the same time, and he feels he has control over his behavior. Kit does not.

### "It's Only Sexual If She Wants It to Be"

A man's awareness of the level on which he is operating, as we have seen, does not necessarily preclude him from sexually offensive behavior. This mode of boundary monitoring is most problematic when men put out a message at Level A but decide that it's up to the woman to decide whether the sexual element is there. Gary exemplifies this attitude when he says, "And even though I can talk to her in a way that doesn't *seem* sexual, I look for any sign that she is taking it sexually, because if she wants it to be, then it is."

It's as if the sexuality in his message were being held out as bait: If a woman doesn't take the bait by engaging in sexual communication, the man can claim that his behavior was nonsexual; if she takes the bait by responding at a sexual level, it becomes *her* responsibility for sexualizing matters.

There is an obvious flaw in this traditionally masculine boundary-testing strategy: The man fails to take responsibility for having initially sexualized the boundary interaction. But a potentially more dangerous flaw involves the masculine tendency to read sexuality into a woman's response when it is not there at all. Steve Horner, for example, was unable to accurately read Sally Dunheim's responses to his request for a "real kiss" because he had decided that her earlier responses indicated sexual interest. As he subsequently discovered, he was totally wrong about this; on the contrary, she had experienced his request for a kiss as unwelcome sexual behavior, the very stuff of sexual harassment.

### Men and Inaccurate "Reads"

The tendency of men to come up with inaccurate "reads" of women's boundary experiences is one of the factors that gives the most trouble in male-female boundary behaviors, both in and outside the workplace. The fact that these inaccuracies are likely to veer in the direction of finding sexual interest in a woman's behavior when there is none is dangerous, because they can lead to boundary violations that run the spectrum from mildly offensive behavior to persistent harassment, even to stalking and rape.

An attorney once sent me a client who had an extreme case of thinking "When she says no, she means yes" about a woman at work of whom he was enamored. He had agreed to counseling in return for a minor reprimand on his work record and an agreement that he stay away from the object of his desires thereafter. But no matter what the woman did, he kept misreading her behavior as a sign that she was attracted to him. When he first began counseling with me, he was certain that even her sexual harassment complaint was an encoded signal of her interest in him, and he saw it as his mission to persist in the heroic quest of winning her hand. Fortunately, he was not a violent man, and he proved open to examining this fantasy as a way of understanding more about himself. Still, it took more than a year of work, exploring the meaning of his fantasy and learning how to read communication better, before he let her go.

It is also important to recognize that boundary testing can be occurring even when the person doing the testing does not identify what he is doing as flirting. Some men's flirtatiousness is so intrinsic to their normal relational style that they can touch women, make double-entendre jokes, and comment copiously on women's looks, then honestly proclaim, "But that's just *me!*"

As discussed here, persistent boundary-testing behavior is the outward manifestation of managing boundaries from misread cues. The psychological reasons underlying such behavior, which involve the ways in which men use their sexual fantasies, are covered at greater length in the next chapter.

### Feminine Boundary Strategies

Sexual boundary and harassment problems cannot be avoided simply because men are confident that they know the difference between Levels A and B. It is also essential that they consider the way that the women in their environment experience *them.* This perception is new for many men; until it was legally articulated in 1991 in the *Ellison v. Brady* Reasonable Woman decision, the "experience of women" had been systematically excluded from the way in which our society determined the welcomeness of sexual boundary behavior.

Rebecca, a woman in her mid-twenties who reluctantly sued her employer in the insurance industry, told me her story:

> I was brought up in a community with very traditional values, where I was told you could trust other people's common decency. I worked hard, thought I was doing well, and counted on its being appreciated. But my boss just kept hitting on me to go out with him. He was married, I never showed him any interest, and I brought my boyfriend around to work.
>
> But one night he starts telling me that he hopes my boyfriend treats me right, and that if *he* were my boyfriend, he would do thus and so to please me. I just freaked. I started screaming, left

work, and never went back. I was once really enthusiastic about working. Now it makes me sick to even think of being in an office alone with a man again.

Was this a "reasonable" response for Rebecca to have had? Recall that Judge Beezer spoke to this question when he wrote, "Women who are victims of mild forms of sexual harassment may understandably worry whether a harasser's conduct is merely a prelude to violent sexual assault. Men . . . may view sexual conduct . . . without a full appreciation of the social setting or the underlying threat of violence that a woman may perceive."

Even when a man feels he is operating on safe and proper Level A— behaving in ways he feels are not sexual—some of what he does may be experienced as sexual by the women around him. The so-called "nonsexual" neck rubs that Ed gave Winnie are a good example. A woman can well experience the "underlying threat of violence" that Judge Beezer mentions when her boundaries are sexualized in ways that are far from violent but that are unwelcome. Once when I was consulting with a group of younger women food service workers who were discussing harassment, a woman described a so-called "dumb blonde" joke, told by a man in her workplace. It referred to a woman allegedly enjoying sex with an entire football team. Uniformly, the women in the group were not only offended by the "joke" but sickened and scared. "Yuck, that's weird!" was one response. The man who had told the joke had not been violent; nor had he been "coming on" to any woman in particular. Yet almost all the women had a gut-level reaction of fear to the allusion to sexual violence in the "joke."

### Women and the Sense of Place

In what different ways do women monitor sexual boundaries as they work and play alongside men? While men monitor for sexual possibilities, I believe that women monitor primarily for a sense of *place*. If a man's sexual monitoring sometimes reflects an anxiety that can be alleviated by sexual interest, a woman's concern about place reflects an insecurity about whether she will be seen to belong at work at all. This insecurity is understandable in the light of the long historical exclusion of women from the workplace and from public life. Yet I believe that even outside the work setting, women monitor boundaries for a sense of their place in a world whose rules have for the most part been constructed without including "the experience of women."

What is meant by monitoring for a sense of place? Primarily, it means a woman's watching the boundaries of her relationships with others for feeling states that might threaten her place, and also (as described earlier in this chapter) trying to mend disharmonies when they occur. Much of the priority a woman gives to monitoring these feeling states, I sense, is based on her need to keep alert to anything that would threaten her feeling that she *belongs* where she is.

Mary, an account executive at a stock brokerage firm, explained the feminine approach to boundaries in this way:

> You know, I feel very confident about what I do. I don't think my job performance is judged any differently from the way it is for men, and I usually come out near the top. So I know I've earned my place here. But you'd have to be completely oblivious not to know that lots of people don't feel the same way.
>
> They see a woman at work at what used to be a man's job, and something goes off in them because I'm a *woman*, instead of because I'm *me*, a good broker. I feel this as a level of tension with the mostly male brokers and customers I deal with every day. If I make a mistake, suddenly it will be because I'm a woman.
>
> You can't change the attitude of everyone around you, and I don't try. I wouldn't say I'm subservient or even especially diplomatic if men get upset with me. I just try to move on from it. But I can never escape the reality that, if someone is unhappy with me, I may be seen not just as a lousy stockbroker but as a damn woman who shouldn't have been trying to do this in the first place. I don't think about always proving my competence to others, since I feel secure in it myself. But I must admit that when they post the monthly numbers and mine happen to be at the top, I get a special satisfaction, because at that moment I'm a broker, not a *woman* broker.
>
> But that doesn't last very long. In all of my interactions with people, I'm aware of the potential for them to shift at any time

to seeing me as a woman first. So if a guy begins to flirt, it's almost always a burden. It's one more thing I have to try to manage and not let bad feelings get going. Especially if it's a customer, I've got to walk that fine line between, in his eyes, not being a bitch, a lesbian, a whore, and just plain not hurting his feelings. Not that I particularly care how he sees me, but my job does depend on it.

It's not that I'm shut down sexually at work—on the rare occasion that someone interesting comes along and it doesn't threaten my work, I can feel attracted to someone. But there's not much room to dwell on that, and I don't want to feed that energy. I know some guys are thinking about it all the time, but why do they bother? If some sexual connection happens, it happens. Eventually it probably will, and you deal with it then.

### The Burden of Sexualized Messages

Mary's attitude demonstrates several important elements of the feminine approach to boundaries. First and most important, she is clearly overloaded with trying to manage people's attitudes toward her because she is a woman. Although inwardly she feels entitled to her place, she can't shut down the way others around her feel. Her attitude also demonstrates that monitoring boundaries for harmony rather than for sex does not mean that women are nurturing or more emotional; Mary's way of dealing with boundaries seems like a reasonable, strategic approach rather than a caretaking one.

Something else that Mary's experience demonstrates is how disruptive it is for women when men introduce a sexual element into the relationship. I wouldn't characterize Mary as oversensitive, hysterical, or even threatened by a man who creates a sexual boundary event. But she clearly does not appreciate it, would much rather do without it, and finds it discouraging each time it happens.

Like many women, Mary couldn't even survive at work without possessing a high tolerance for dealing with a great many day-to-day sexual boundary events. One senses that she would not take well to a man who didn't "get it" and persisted in his sexual behavior despite her lack of interest. Yet Mary's high priority of maintaining and solidifying her place at work is typical of women who try to manage sexual boundary behavior on their own rather than pursue a sexual harassment complaint.

Hence, women are less likely to be receptive to sexualized Level B behavior from men. What they appreciate most is men not creating sexual boundary events. As Mary has suggested, relax, guys—enough sexual events will happen without pushing so hard to make them happen. Dalia seemed to have a reasonable formula in mind:

> It's so easy to ask a woman at work out, really. Just take it real slow. Ask us to lunch first, and talk about work. If we say no the next two times, forget it completely. If we say yes or ask you to lunch, just stick with the lunches for a couple of weeks, but hang back about putting too much personal stuff into the conversation. After about three months, ask us to dinner. If we say yes, then you've really crossed the boundary to making it personal. But you've always got to be ready to let it go when we tell you it's enough. And none of that jokey-flirty stuff at work, either. It's not necessary, and it's a turn-off.

To include the other gender's experience in your boundary feedback loop is to take a huge step forward. When Ed gives Winnie a neck rub, he doesn't see it as sexual because to him it is a Level A act; he is not pulling out the big guns of Level B behavior. But it shouldn't be so difficult for him to understand that Winnie might feel that a neck rub from a man at work, whom she hardly knows, is a sexual boundary event.

Obviously, many women are as involved in sexual boundary monitoring and intrigue as men typically are and, whether at work or elsewhere, are quite adept at sexualizing their interactions with men. A woman named Josie once admitted to me that she had had affairs with several of the men at work and was known as the "office tramp." In fact, at one point she had been quite proud of her open sexuality, but she was now having second thoughts after one of her co-workers, who didn't interest her, had given her a lift home and had nearly raped her when she didn't give him his anticipated sexual payment.

Nonetheless, my sense is that there have never been as many sexually available women as men have thought or hoped there were; this is part of the masculine tendency to read sexuality into women's behavior when there is none. In a great many cases, the sexually seductive woman is a fantasy creation of men, although there are certainly many women who attempt to adapt to what they think men want. Nevertheless, when women are at work, even those who might fit the cultural stereotype of the sexy, seductive woman are showing less tolerance for the notion that their dress, speech, and body language justify unwelcome sexual behavior.

Laura's story is a good example. Her attorney told me that Laura was suing her boss at a credit bureau for harassment because he developed a trick of dropping a piece of paper, then asking her to pick it up while he stared down her neckline. In the investigation of the harassment charge, it came out that half of the women in the office had witnessed this behavior and had been outraged at its flagrance. But a few women, and many of the men, were prepared to testify in her boss's favor because, as some of them put it, "She is the sexiest thing to come into our office in years, and she does nothing to hide it."

Outrage at the boss's behavior is the attitude that represents the future of our ability to assess certain types of sexual behavior. But the attitude of those who supported the boss represents the past: that if a woman is "sexy" in the eyes of certain beholders, she is responsible for bringing on whatever kinds of sexual behavior are directed toward her.

### Different Boundary Agendas, Common Ground

When you place the Level B sexual agenda of men next to the agenda of women, it looks as if the sexes are working at cross purposes. But in many ways the gulf between these two agendas is not that huge. Men too are looking for a sense of place, but they attempt to get it through sexuality; likewise, women can get to sexuality through a sense of place. Rafe, the health care industry CEO who had worked so hard to resist his sexual fantasizing about his boss, was able to find his sense of place in creative work and a healthy relationship that included sexuality. And Barbara, the computer programmer who developed a relationship with her co-worker Nate, had no trouble eventually allowing the relationship to become sexual, once she realized that it did not threaten her sense of place. As she saw it, "If Nate had moved too fast to make things sexual, it would have scared me off, because I really wanted to keep working and would have resented his making me feel split between being a worker and being a woman. If a guy knows how to respect both things in us at the same time, I think that workplace romance is more feasible than most people think. But if you meet at work, he has to go *really* slow with the sexual agenda."

I believe that the differences in how men and women sequence their quests for sexual intimacy and a sense of place are due to their longtime socialization into completely different cultural expectations. When our culture finally grants women an equal place with men and dissuades men from attempts at sexual coercion, both genders will have more room, if they choose, to experience sexuality at work as laden with interesting possibilities, rather than as a burden and a threat. At the same time, as the culture supplies men with new role models for creative containment of their sexuality, replacing the old role models that lionize those who are adept at crossing sexual boundaries, a sense of masculine place can emerge without its needing sexual validation from women. When I was working with Rafe, he told me, "You're the first man I ever talked to about my sexual fantasies who told me that they were about *me*, not about *her*."

We all want to have a safe and meaningful sense of belonging, and most people also long for sexual intimacy that is integrated not only in a relationship but in their place in the world. Women and men actually have a great deal in common. As we realize this, we can also look forward to what might at first seem like a paradox but isn't really one at all: the *sexually* Reasonable Woman and Man.

## FLIRTING AND BOUNDARY TESTING

Having defined the fundamental difference between male and female attitudes toward *monitoring* boundary events, let's take a more detailed look at the way in which men and women behave in the subsequent boundary stages.

The next step is *boundary testing.* A key means of boundary testing is flirting. Through flirting, a timeless, universal human signaling system, people send and receive information that, at its best, helps them sort out what is occurring at the sexual boundary. But what to one person is flirting can be unwelcome sexual behavior to another, so flirting deserves close scrutiny if we are to understand and prevent sexual harassment—or offensive boundary behavior of any kind.

Although many sexual harassment scenarios occur because of differences between men and women's understanding of flirting, there are actually many points of agreement between the sexes on the subject. After all, no information signaling system would work if those involved didn't agree on some of the meanings it encodes.

Most people realize that sexual interest is signaled in a variety of ways: through different kinds of speaking, whether tone of voice or choice of words; through glances, facial expressions, and the management of the critical parameter of eye contact; through physical positioning; through timing, often expressed as holding a handshake for an extra moment, or by lingering just a bit longer when any particular social interaction is about to end; through pace of interaction (asking someone to lunch three days running sends a different message than having lunch once a week for three weeks); through phone calls, conversations, notes, cards, gifts, semiarranged "just running into's," or just about any way of initiating or sustaining communication.

None of the above is a problem as long as both people involved are willing participants and have a fairly similar grasp of the rules. Once again, the critical skill involved here is the ability to monitor the feedback loop accurately. When you ask someone to lunch and he or she accepts for three days running, you still cannot really know with certainty whether the person is just being polite within the workplace context. If that person turns around and suggests you have dinner together next week, it sends one message. If he or she continues treating you politely but with no further mention of lunches, you're in limbo. But if that person no longer stops to exchange a few words when you pass in the hall and keeps on having other plans for lunch when you ask again, it's disappointing but extremely important to accept the information being conveyed. Both Barbara and Dalia recommend going "real slow," not being opportunistic, and recognizing, as Dalia adds, "In all circumstances, no means no. I can't think of a more depressing, destructive, and wrong-headed stereotype than that when we women put up barriers, it's because we want men to try harder to knock them down. I don't know what century that came under, but I wouldn't want to have lived then, and the twenty-first century is going to be different."

What all acts of flirting have in common is that they convey something extra that exceeds the already-established context of the situation. That something extra is an act of boundary testing. Once you accept that any act of flirting is also an act of boundary testing, and begin to understand how complex are the assumptions behind even innocent or appropriate flirting, it is easy to see where the many pitfalls lie.

Great powers of discernment need to be put to use even before that critical first act of flirting is attempted. Because flirting is boundary testing and exceeds what is required by the workplace context, two judgments are needed from the start: (1) What exactly *is* the agreed-upon context? and (2) Does that context have any room for even a low-profile, initial act of flirting? Chapter 5 presents detailed suggestions about how to deal with these questions.

## BOUNDARY RESPECTING

One factor that clearly differentiates characteristic male and female boundary behavior is men's almost automatic Level B involvement when they interact with women who interest them. As noted, there is nothing amiss in itself in this sexual fantasizing. Rafe's story is an instructional account of how even a reasonable man can be driven half-crazy with sexual fantasy, yet can gain from the ordeal if he is able to protect his boundary behavior from turning into a vehicle for his fantasy life.

"How could I ever have found out what was *inside* if I kept acting it out *outside?*" Rafe told me. "Once you get past the almost addictive compulsion to touch this or that woman, you realize that you have your own inner strength that you've never drawn upon. That lively quality that we're attracted to in the woman can actually be found inside. And until I found it, I felt that I was involved in this childlike dependency, even if I could mask it with somewhat aggressive male behavior."

Boundary respecting is an important option in boundary behavior. But what is so unfortunate, and demeaning to men as well as women, is that many men have been raised in a culture that considers a failure to follow up on sexual fantasy with action to be "unmanly." The model of "playing games" and trying to "score" is sometimes so built into a man's psychology that he habitually approaches all interactions with women from this framework.

Besides constantly barraging women with sexualized behavior, men following this model can have a seriously impaired feedback loop. A strong current in men's psychology tells them that when they encounter an obstacle—in this case a boundary—they must push ever more strongly against it. This is why even when women give fairly clear notice about their lack of interest, some men regard it as a challenge to be overcome. If a woman says no three times straight to having lunch, for example, it is a gross misreading of boundaries for a man to call her at home in the evening and ask her to have dinner, to send her flowers, or to write her notes telling her how special she is.

As we have noted, much of the persistent drive that impels men to escalate their boundary-crossing behavior despite discouraging feedback comes from their sexual fantasy lives. As long as society sanctions this kind of escalation, men will not be encouraged to learn to contain their fantasies and will continue to try to play them out regardless of their appropriateness. Developing the concept of boundary respecting, a legitimate and respectable option *not* to engage in flirting or boundary testing of any kind, helps clarify new directions in male psychology.

As Judge Beezer said in his Reasonable Woman decision, "Conduct considered harmless by many today may be considered discriminatory in the future. . . . As the views of reasonable women [and men] change, so too does the Title VII standard of acceptable behavior." I have taken the liberty of inserting "and men" into this quotation because I believe that one thing being asked of men is that they learn to *internalize* these new standards of boundary behavior, rather than put their women co-workers and human resources officers in the position of policing their behavior. This is yet another way in which the Reasonable Man joins the Reasonable Woman in solving sexual boundary problems.

# 4. SEXUAL FANTASIES

## *How Inner Life Affects Outer Boundaries*

Seated together at her desk in the marketing department, Linda and Tom look over the memo to the vice-president that they have prepared proposing an entirely new way of promoting InfoTech's hot new communications software package. When Tom performs a mild impression of their boss reading the memo, Linda laughs and grasps Tom's right forearm with her left hand for a full three seconds.

In that brief span, Tom's entire world suddenly shifts. He has seen the brainy Linda as an interesting but sexless co-worker "buddy" for the three months they have been working together on this project. But with that three-second arm grasp, he realizes that Linda's abundant energy and talent for creating memos with him has transformed itself into a powerful desire on her part to go to bed with him. Because they are on a deadline, he maintains his outer cool as they deliver the memo and rush off to separate meetings. But that evening after work, Tom fantasizes everything from a sexual encounter with Linda at her desk to a weekend tryst in his condo to a life together.

Meanwhile, as Linda pulls her hand back from Tom's arm, she fantasizes about the promotion and raise that this near-perfect memo could bring her. Never in her ten-year career in the high-tech industry has she felt the creative buzz she feels with Tom. She realizes that she likes him immensely and marvels at having teamed up creatively with a man who, during three months of cheek-by-jowl work together, often alone in the office after hours, has sent her not even a smidgen of a sexual vibe.

As they deliver the memo and rush off to their meetings, she thanks her lucky stars that she works with Tom, and she tries to suppress the memory of the countless male co-workers who couldn't wait two days, much less two weeks, before ruining their working relationship with a sexualized move or comment.

The next day Tom comes to work feeling euphoric, ready to let the boundaries down at the next opportune "signal" from Linda.

No matter how many sexual harassment laws a society enacts, or how conscious each of us becomes about sexual boundary behavior, there will always be moments of special, overwhelming impact when we feel an instant sexual or love connection for someone. Whether we attribute them to love potions, bewitchments, metaphorical arrows shot through the heart, or other divine interventions, these moments of instantaneous erotic fantasy-awakening are the stuff of poetry, drama, art, and song. They can be laced with beauty and touch our innermost yearnings—or they can go astray, unleashing a destructive power that generates divisiveness where we work, torment in our homes, and even violence.

What is more, we cannot anticipate such erotic moments. They come upon us unbidden, without regard for time or place: on the street, on a bus, driving down the road; at home with friends, at a party, in a dorm, on a check-out line, in a restaurant, in a house of worship; and of course, where we work or learn: in the office, the classroom, the library, or passing each other in the hallway.

To be sure, not all moments of fantasy awakening have such magical or formidable power. Their shape and intensity vary; some fantasies are private dalliances that last no more than a few minutes or perhaps hours, then ebb of their own accord or are replaced by the next fantasy stimulus. But intense or not, the power of sexual fantasy in its most magical, fully developed form is always within us, capable of coming into play at any time.

As Oliver, a thirty-two-year-old single man who had just begun a job as a high school English teacher, put it, "Every day's a marvelous adventure for my fantasies. I get to review them all when I get home and then see what I'll dream of at night. Last week, just a glance from Valerie in my senior class set me spinning with pleasure for the day. But yesterday she was replaced by Moira, who wrote this terrific paper that made me want to stay up half the night with her talking about literature and the soul. I fall in love with each of them in a different way." Fortunately, Oliver is an ethical man who knows he should not act on these fantasies—but there are times when he has been tempted. His description of the capacity to form instant, magical fantasy connections sheds light on the dynamics that motivate inappropriate outer boundary crossings.

## VARIETIES OF SEXUAL FANTASY

As Oliver implies, fantasies vary in their content. Some are frankly sexual in form, bringing us an instant imagining of actual physical coupling. Others involve the creation of a psychological and emotional connection as well, through conversations, gazes into each other's eyes, walks, journeys, and other shared activities, with or without sexual contact. Fantasies can be highly spiritualized, with inner states of awakening and transcendence interweaving with or taking precedence over the sexual. Sadly, once we enter the fantasy world, as in the dream world, we may be unable to keep our fantasies from turning dark and visiting us with images of suffering, grief, and violence—even sexual violence.

Every one of us has an invisible inner dimension, a full-spectrum sexual fantasy life that lies behind the dimensions we are aware of. Just as we can learn to decode the outward signals of flirting and boundary-testing behavior, we can also come to understand the more mysterious workings of the inner fantasy world.

In this chapter we will examine the dynamics of these special and not-so-special fantasies, and their relationship to boundary problems and sexual harassment. We'll take a more detailed look at what occurred between Tom and Linda, and *inside* Tom and Linda, in the three seconds that she touched his arm. For you, such moments may have taken a different form: the briefest of gazes or smiles or gestures, a few words exchanged, or a voice over the telephone—just enough for you to imagine that the other person is also interested in you. Or perhaps the individual in your fantasy was entirely unaware of your existence—you saw him or her "across a crowded room," in a photograph, on stage or screen, or in a dating service dossier: a fantasy object who never even knew of your imaginings. Ultimately, the person who can set off this flood of hope or passion, of sexual desire or spiritual vision, need do nothing at all except make an entrance into your life.

It is ironic that the most likely places for fantasy triggers today are the very arenas where our sexual boundary behavior is now most closely scrutinized and regulated: at work and at school. This irony has a positive aspect, however. Given the misunderstandings and outright disasters that come from mishandling powerful erotic feelings, codes of conduct at work and on campus should be welcome, not for their punitive possibilities but because in raising our awareness of how we handle our sexual boundaries, they can help us avert catastrophe.

In pointing this out, I am not trying to pour cold water on the special moments that trigger these intense fantasies. When they are mutual, they can sometimes have a raw energy that enables the two people to transform their relationship into a real and enduring one. But a full-blown fantasy scenario resting wholly in one person's mind can impel that person to cross over boundaries in ways that are sexually harassing, and even dangerous.

## FANTASIES AS INFORMATION ABOUT WHAT IS WITHIN US

Although the way some people use fantasy can at times drive them toward boundary-violating behavior, fantasies themselves are part of a rich and resourceful psychological world from which new solutions can emerge for old problems. The balance between conscious awareness and unconsciousness can actually support the healthy integration into our lives of the beauty promised in our fantasies. But to allow that balance to develop, we must recognize how our management of boundaries and fantasies affects those around us. In fact, the balancing force for a sexual boundary crisis can sometimes emerge from a fantasy or a dream.

Jeff was propelled into a sudden, all-consuming fantasy about a woman who looked into his eyes in a way that, as he put it, "captured eternity." Full of excitement, he decided to show up on her doorstep and proclaim his undying love for her. The night before this planned encounter, he dreamed that he was trying to get on a train to visit her. The old man in the ticket booth gave him not a ticket but a small leather pouch filled with small stones. He woke up feeling that the old man in the booth was somehow right to bar him from trying to live out his fantasy, and he decided to put off visiting her. Although this saddened him, he also felt that the stones represented reality—and he found he was glad to be able to "ground" his fantasy. It was a very good thing he did—he was her psychotherapist, and it would have been a catastrophic boundary violation for both of them if he had proceeded.

Tom, in the energized office meeting described at the beginning of this chapter, is faced with a similar challenge. At the fantasy level, he is sure that Linda's three-second arm touch is a Level B sexual signal to him. Can he, or anyone in his position, learn how to manage such a fantasy internally, so that it does not guide his boundary behavior? It is not easy to develop the ability to create an internal boundary for a sexual fantasy, but the rewards reach beyond the mere avoidance of harassing behavior; it can help enhance an individual's integrity and capacity for appropriate intimacy.

## STAGES IN MEN'S MANAGEMENT OF SEXUAL FANTASIES

Just as the management of sexual boundaries has definable stages, the development and management of sexual fantasies has stages. These stages are *fantasy formation, exploration, testing,* and *resolution.* Each has a corresponding effect on sexual boundary behavior. And as in boundary behavior, the stages that women experience may be similar to those for men, but their characteristic ways of managing each stage are quite different.

Let's look at the effect on Tom of Linda's touch on his arm. The initial stage, *fantasy formation,* goes into play the moment he feels her touch. But a sexual response often launches men quite rapidly into the next stage, *fantasy exploration.* Linda's touch sends Tom almost completely into his fantasy world. Although the actual touch on the arm means very little to her, Tom, within a few seconds of its occurrence, is inwardly exploring some major issues of his life: sexuality, companionship, and detailed scenarios of a rosy future, all to be shared with Linda.

It is important to emphasize that there is nothing inherently pathological about Tom's response, or about any man spending hours or even days thinking about the meaning of three seconds of a woman's actions toward him. Ultimately, boundary and sexual harassment problems are defined by our *behavior*, even when they are strongly pressured by our fantasies. No matter how preoccupied we may be with a fantasy, we remain responsible for staying aware of social reality—and for acting appropriately toward others. This responsibility can be difficult to carry out. Whenever sexuality is involved, there is a danger that men, to a far greater degree than women, will behave in ways that try to gratify the fantasy.

Innumerable fantasy scenarios lie waiting in a man's psyche, ready to be triggered by the mere presence of a woman, at times not requiring even a hint of a smile or other cues from her. Indeed, in its pure form, the triggering female presence comes without anyone being there at all, in a daydream or night dream. Nevertheless, as long as a man maintains an inner constraint against acting on the basis of fantasy, his outward boundary behavior need not reflect his inner preoccupation.

### Testing Sexual Fantasy Through Imposition

It is at the next stage of fantasy development, *fantasy testing*, that the most troublesome element of male boundary behavior enters the picture. Unless men are able to maintain their inner constraint, they may attempt to impose the structure of their fantasy onto others.

This imposition can show itself through a whole range of sexual behaviors, from sexual bantering all the way to stalking and rape. In fact, some of the more common forms of sexual harassment—sexual comments, sexual jokes, and the posting of erotic pictures—are all interrelated ways in which men bring their fantasy lives into daily public behavior.

"Whew, it's hot," a warehouse worker said to his woman trainee one afternoon. "When we get off shift, let's take a nice shower together back at the dispatching center." "Hey, babe, if you get tired of that chair, you can just sit on me" went a comment from a male office worker to a woman at a desk near his. A woman carpenter asked a man on her crew if she could use the hammer on his belt. "Sure, but I've got a tool you'd really like under the belt," he replied.

Although comments like these are often considered "normal" sexual banter, these men are actually presenting their sexual fantasies and asking women to step into them. Problems can readily occur when the woman in a man's sex-tinged fantasy does not play her expected part. Before sexual harassment law, the male practice of posting erotic and even frankly pornographic pictures of women in the workplace not only went unchallenged but was considered a norm. Through these images, men kept their sexual fantasy lives fueled while at work.

A crucial moment of decision occurs when a man gets an inkling that his fantasy is not appreciated, much less shared, by the woman he is fantasizing about. In which direction will he turn when he perceives a conflict between his inner wish and the outer reality? Will he work even harder to bring about the outcome he desires—or will he be able to retreat and contain his fantasy?

No matter how deeply influenced men may be by evolutionary biology, by hormones, or by previous social training and sex-role spillover to push toward realizing their sexual fantasies, society is now asking them to learn new ways of managing their yearnings. This is the moment when men most need to step out of the past and to respect the new standards that have been created by sexual harassment law.

Of signal importance among these new standards is men's responsibility to avoid any sexual speech or behavior toward women in the workplace that could reasonably be experienced as unwelcome, a position strongly articulated in the *Ellison v. Brady* Reasonable Woman decision. The sexual harassment scenario that led to this decision involved a man imposing his fantasy on a woman. As we have seen, one of the notes the male co-worker in this case wrote to Kerry Ellison read:

> I have enjoyed you so much over these past few months. Watching you. Experiencing you from O so far away. Admiring your style and elan. . . . Don't you think it odd that two people who have never even talked together, alone, are striking off such intense sparks. . . . I will [write] another letter in the near future.

There seems little doubt that this man was seeing not Ellison, but a woman in his own fantasy life. Unfortunately, at moments like this, when a man most needs to use his "reasonable" side to distinguish between inner and outer, many factors are working against reason. Conflict between a fantasy scenario and the outer reality creates strong feelings that are not usually considered reasonable. Depending on his individual emotional makeup, a man's feelings upon discovering that his fantasy is not turning into reality can run the gamut from anxiety, anger, and depression to denial and despair at the impending loss. Thus, men must do their best—that is, deal reasonably with the discrepancy between fantasy and reality—at the very moment when they may be at their emotional worst. Nevertheless, it is necessary for all of us, regardless of gender, to do precisely this, in order to live up to ethical and legal standards that society asks of us.

## WOMEN'S MANAGEMENT OF THEIR FANTASIES

Linda, for her part, has also to come to terms with the fantasy that was awakened in her during that fateful office meeting when she touched Tom's arm. Although not sexually charged, her fantasy is passionate in its own way, and she faces a similar challenge of trying to integrate the reality of who Tom is with the person her inner world wishes him to be. For women as well as men, the person they imagine someone to be in their fantasies is likely to be at odds with who the person really is.

Women's development of fantasy can be divided into the same stages as men's—fantasy formation, exploration, testing, and resolution. Men's and women's ways of managing fantasy have other similarities as well: For all of us, the fantasy world is a place where we can experience a meeting between what is outside us and what is within us, a place where we can allow ourselves to think and feel whatever we wish about others, about how they are treating us, about who we are, and about our most horrible fears and our most cherished hopes. Fantasy at its best can also bring the external world inside us so that we can work out imaginative and creative ways to adapt to that world, while at the same time satisfy our longing for safety, intimacy, and a sense of purpose.

As she and Tom review the memo they have prepared together, Linda too experiences a powerful fantasy formation, one that, like Tom's, proceeds immediately to an intense fantasy exploration. For her as for him, something suddenly clicks, and she becomes extremely excited about her productive interaction with Tom and all the possibilities it holds for her future. Although she is tracking this initial interaction down a very different path, she is equally moved by it.

## Women's Passionate Nonsexual Fantasies

Linda, while intensely "turned on" by her meeting with Tom, is having a fantasy that is not at all sexual. It's not that women don't have instantaneous sexual fantasies, or that the type of passionate, nonsexual fantasy that she is having cannot quickly evolve into a sexual one. It's just that at this point in our cultural history, there seems to be much more room in the female psyche for a passionate, exciting, and intense fantasy about someone without its being sexual.

This is how it occurs for Linda. Although she touches Tom's arm, no sexual signaling is intended in this touch. While for Tom it triggers overwhelming erotic fantasy, Linda barely notices that she is doing it. At that moment she is carried away by the sheer excitement of the creative potential in the work she and Tom are doing together.

For Linda, as for many women, school and the workplace are settings in which they can awaken to capacities that they may have felt the world would never allow them to fulfill. The onrush of passion that engulfs their fantasies is likely to be motivated by the hope that their entire selves, not just their sexual selves, will have a place in society's public marketplace of work, education, commerce, and politics.

Full involvement for women in these male-dominated realms involves the psychological task—to use Jungian terminology—of developing the animus. It is not that the skills women need in order to function equally with men in the workplace, in the university, in corporate culture, and in public life are *objectively* masculine; it's just that they have been defined as such in our world and assigned by sex-role stereotype to men.

Animus development does not mean becoming masculine. For an individual woman, the animus is a way of identifying strengths in herself that—given permission and support to go beyond sex-role stereotypes—she may move toward developing. Thus, a woman who was brought up to be the family peacemaker and mollify other people's anger might in adulthood find it useful at times to let others know that she is angry with them. If she has been brought up to defer to a man in a relationship and let him drive the car or make family decisions, she might instead become less deferential and "drive the car" more often herself, both literally and metaphorically. The objective of animus development for a woman is not to prove a point or win a power struggle but to become more *herself*, transcending the limitations of who she was told she should be. Dreams and fantasies can help women surmount these limitations. They often involve either an actual man or a purely inner masculine figure who serves as the carrier of the vision, and the raw energy that will enable them to develop parts of themselves that have been neglected.

### Women's Fantasies of Safety: Place Without Sexual Price

At present, women's fantasies are rooted in the hope that the place society accords them will embrace their whole selves, not only their sexual selves; and this is where the fantasy dynamics of women and men seem to be at such cross-purposes. If a woman is to have a sense of place that is truly hers, she must feel that she must pay *absolutely* no sexual price for it. This place is precisely what Linda is exploring in her fantasy. Not only is the fantasy passionate yet nonsexual, but the very absence of sexual pressure, the sense of safety from sexual demand she feels with Tom, is what has allowed her to become so excited.

In fact, this may be part of the reason she touched Tom's arm. Although she scarcely noticed the action and it was not sexual, neither was it done carelessly or without meaning. Her gesture was if anything a sign of closeness and trust, a shared moment with someone whom she respects and appreciates.

It is the breach of this trust that is so devastating for women in school and the workplace: that instant when they discover that a man who has been an important mentor or a valued colleague also has sexual designs on them. At that moment, the heart can go out of all they have put into their jobs or courses of study. An unwelcome sexualizing of a woman's boundary with a man can shatter her fantasy of having a place in the world that is not conditioned upon her sexual availability.

Although most women are savvy enough to realize that many men around them view them sexually, the fact that they expect boundary-testing behavior from men does not mean that they want it, or that it isn't demeaning, depressing, and often harmful. Indeed, most women at work do not expect the degree of safety that Linda hoped for with Tom. Quite the opposite: They report almost universally that they couldn't survive for a single day if they did not learn to cope with a certain level of sexualized behavior from men as a kind of "background noise." Nevertheless, every now and again a woman may renew her hope as Linda did, through a particular man she works with, that there is a safety zone from this constant barrage against her boundaries. It is when even this man sexualizes her boundaries that she loses hope.

## TOM AND LINDA: A BOUNDARY DISASTER TAKING SHAPE

A characteristic and major dividing line runs between men and women in the transition from fantasy exploration to *fantasy testing,* the next stage. The genders have learned very different skills when it comes to expressing what they feel inside.

As we saw in the example of Steve asking Sally for a "real kiss," boundary testing is the stage where most incidents of sexual harassment occur. From the different ways that Tom and Linda are tracking their interaction even before the testing stage begins, a potential disaster is taking shape.

The day after Linda's arm touch and Tom's excited, near-sleepless night thinking about its implications, the two co-workers have another meeting to work on their project. When Tom first walks into Linda's small, enclosed office, all he can see is the glow of the woman on whom he has developed an overwhelming crush. But Tom is not an irresponsible man. Conflicting with the intoxication of his fantasy life is his sense of social propriety and respect for Linda and the workplace.

In this situation, Tom resorts to the standard male behavior of Level A and Level B boundary monitoring. Outwardly, he sits down and tries to pay attention to the draft of the new memo that Linda is showing him. She has added some rough drawings and excitedly points them out to him as they sit close to each other, looking at the material on her desk.

Surprisingly, Tom is able to comprehend the material before him and even respond to it. But inwardly he is intensely monitoring the situation for signs of Linda's erotic interest in him. He feels the faint brushes of her body against him as she positions herself to show him the papers. He senses her energy and enthusiasm. His inward thought stream goes like this: *I can tell she's excited and energized, but is it or isn't it sexual for her? What did she mean by touching my arm yesterday and brushing against me today?*

With that thought, Tom realizes that he's going off track, getting lost in his fantasy again. He refocuses on the project. As they scrutinize the papers in front of them on the desk, Linda is no longer brushing against him. They are now sitting side by side, with two inches of empty space between them. Although they make brief eye contact when they speak to each other, their gaze for the most part is straight down, on the work itself. But now Tom begins to get anxious. He's noticing the absence of erotic signaling from Linda. Although he wasn't expecting anything overtly sexual to occur quite yet, it would have been great to feel just a few more touches, or perhaps even a clearer indication that she mirrors his sexual interest. Anxiety leads to confusion as the signs of her interest that he wishes for do not appear.

Tom is now at that crucial turning point when men either become proactive about testing boundaries, or maintain a more reflective inward stance of respecting them. In an attempt to resolve his confusion, he decides to move to the next stage and test the boundary with Linda for her sexual interest.

For many men, a strong push toward taking action springs from the ways they have been taught to resolve anxiety. Although these behaviors may have some evolutionary and hormonal sources, I believe that what tips the balance is learned from cultural, familial, and peer-group sources. Most quarters of our society accord men prestige for their ability to shape the world around them. In situations of sexual boundary tension, this drive for prestige often translates into active boundary testing, which the man uses to shape his relationship with the woman.

But not always, and not necessarily. Our capacity for conscious, thoughtful reflection is also a property of our biological selves, developed as an evolutionary survival skill. I have seen many men pull up these reflective skills from deep within them, contrary to what their cultural conditioning tells them, and refrain from pushing against sexual boundaries.

### To Cross Over or to Turn Back?
### Searching for a Reflective Containment of Fantasy

Although Tom is a reasonably nice guy with reasonably good access to his reflective mode, he does not draw upon this skill. On the other hand, Oliver, the high school English teacher who fell in frequent fantasy-love with his students, was able to. During the year that he consulted with me,

Oliver had a serious crisis that put him in danger of an inappropriate boundary crossing. He was obsessing again about his student Moira, who had started out more as an intellectual fantasy partner but was now becoming a sexual fantasy object as well. It so happened that this crisis occurred just as Oliver had developed a severe case of writer's block while trying to finish a short story he was writing. I pointed out the possible connection between these events and suggested he imagine how his purely inner Moira might write the next part of his story.

A few weeks later, Oliver reported a real breakthrough. "You know, I never really got it before that these fantasy women are, as you said, purely inner figures. Once I accepted that, the pressure about the fantasy woman in my class decreased, and I was able to draw upon my own imagination to help me finish the story."

Oliver was able to see that his fantasy obsession was really about making contact with a feminine creative force of his own—his anima. To cultivate this creativity, he had to turn toward inward reflection and containment and away from concretizing his fantasy. Our culture needs to make these qualities more available to men through role models that teach and clarify the value of reflection over action in dealing with sexual fantasy.

### The Boundary Is Crossed

Let's return to Tom and Linda, who are still in the midst of their meeting. His judgment somewhat clouded by his fantasy, Tom allows his anxiety to push him in the wrong direction: He makes the fateful mistake of moving into the action mode. Still tingling from yesterday's three-second touch on his arm, Tom reciprocates; he places his hand on Linda's thigh.

He rests his hand on her thigh only briefly, but it is long enough to give her an opportunity to show whether she appreciates it by, say, leaning her shoulder toward him and making body contact in return. His hand is on her thigh amply long for Linda to realize that the touch is not inadvertent. It is not at all welcome.

She handles the situation as deftly as she can at the moment—she disengages by rising from her chair, walking a few steps away, and announcing in as pleasantly businesslike a voice as she can muster that she suddenly remembers she has to prepare for another meeting. Externally, they both preserve a semblance of professional demeanor—Tom takes the hint and makes a quick exit from Linda's office. But psychologically, each is falling to pieces. He knows immediately that something is terribly wrong, and that he stands to lose not only his fantasy but possibly his job. Linda remains in her office, but as soon as the door is closed, she collapses into tears, her head buried in her arms on the desk.

## LOSING HEART: BACK TO BUSINESS AS USUAL

When a man she has counted on to be nonsexual discloses his sexual agenda to a woman, the heart can go out of what she is doing at work or at school. This doesnt mean that she will leave or will stop doing what she is there to do. She simply makes an inward adjustment to a more depressing "business as usual" world. She may maintain a pleasant stance, as both Sally and Linda did at the moment their boundaries were crossed, suppress her anger and disappointment, and try to make the best of it. She may also express her anger and sense of insult through protests ranging from direct confrontation to a harassment charge. But whatever course she chooses, she is reminded of how pervasive is the world of old sexual stereotypes—a world that is very far from the ideal of the Reasonable Woman and Reasonable Man working equally together. The reason for Linda's tears, when Tom leaves the room after his unwelcome touch, is that her hope for a new kind of relationship, one that so excited her and stimulated her creativity, is now lying in ruins.

The night before this meeting, Linda also fantasized—about all the creative possibilities for promoting InfoTech's communications software package. Indeed, she got so wrapped up in *her* fantasy that she actually began to think about changes that could be made in the user interface design for the next upgrade of the software itself. Software design is well outside her job description in promotion and sales; she surprised even herself when she discovered that her fantasy was carrying her into a new creative area. Her discovery that new capacities inside herself were pushing her into realms thought of as masculine is another example of the concept of animus development.

## WOMEN'S CAPACITY TO SUSTAIN RATHER THAN TEST FANTASIES

We have seen in Tom and Linda's story the emergence of damaging cross-purposes when women's fantasies of nonsexual safety arise at the same time that men's fantasies are sexualized. Another prominent difference between men's and women's handling of their fantasies is evident at the transition point between fantasy exploration and fantasy testing.

Women, whose fantasies are much more likely to be nonsexual, often do not move on to fantasy testing simply because they have nothing further to test for. The relationship as it already exists has led to the formation of the fantasy, and all that is necessary to test it is to continue the relationship *without* challenging its boundaries.

This means that women can remain in the fantasy-exploration stage for long periods of time. They continue to monitor whether the fantasy can continue to live on in reality. For Linda, this monitoring would have meant further developing her working relationship with Tom without sexual boundaries becoming an issue, and exploring wherever the creative excitement led them. Such nonsexual, creative relationships between men and women in the workplace, are valuable and hopeful new models for our society. On rare occasions, working relationships like these do eventually lead to a sexual connection. But if such a relationship is to develop without destroying a woman's sense of place and safety, it must do so in a completely different way from the stereotypical boundary testing that women experience from men.

At times, of course, women's fantasies are sexualized, but even then they are less likely to test their fantasies through sexual boundary behavior. This is one of the fundamental differences in social sex-role behavior between men and women. Because women tend to monitor the interconnecting relationships around them in an effort to keep them in balance, even if they are sexually interested in a man, they experience less pressure to "make something happen." They are more likely to wait to see whether a sexual connection occurs in a way that does not upset the balance of the relational field around them. Men may misinterpret this, seeing it as a sexual passivity that is waiting for them to engage in more explicit sexual boundary testing. The truth is otherwise. Many women appreciate a man who is able to align himself with a broader relational network and sacrifice his boundary testing.

Karen, a psychologist friend of mine, had just become engaged to Fred, a fellow faculty member at the graduate school where she was teaching. "You know," she told me, "I was fascinated by Fred while I was still a student at the school, and I wondered if he was also attracted to me. But he showed no special interest, so I kind of gave up on that fantasy. Actually, I'm glad he didn't ask me out then because it would have created an enormous ethical mess in the department, which had been notorious for student-professor affairs, all of which turned out badly. But once I finished the program and got hired to teach, there he was. He told me that he *had* been interested in me when I was a student but had resisted doing anything about it. It's such a relief for me to have connected to a man with that kind of integrity."

## FANTASY RESOLUTION: DIFFERENCES BETWEEN MEN AND WOMEN

If it is not disrupted by an unwelcome incursion on their boundaries, fantasy resolution for women can be a purely internal experience. They tend to have more patience for allowing the fantasy to work itself out over time. If a man remains the object of a woman's fantasy, she may simply live with it in a way that is never completely resolved, yet allows her to explore other feelings that relate to her own animus rather than the man himself. These feelings can range from creative passion, such as Linda felt with Tom, to a wide range of emotions such as sexuality, connection, isolation, a sense of threat or safety, anger, sadness, and hope.

I believe that men too have a capacity for internal resolution of their fantasies—it's just that the culture does not support their making use of it. Behind men's tendency to sexualize exciting meetings with women is their potential to explore an inner masculine world from which our society has turned them away, burdening them instead with stereotyped notions of their "real" selves. It is no accident that a man's inner world suddenly opens up when a woman in his environment smiles at him in just the right way. But this sense of enhanced aliveness he is seeking lies within rather than in the hands of the woman who touched off his fantasy. Although there are many different conceptual frameworks for describing how men can accomplish this, much can be understood through the Jungian idea of anima development.

When Oliver was able to give up the outer Moira and draw upon his inner world, it opened up far more in him than the ability to complete his short story successfully. Simply knowing he had done it on one occasion gave him faith in his own inner resources, resources that eventually helped him endure other crises of loss before he found his way to an enduring marriage and a productive life as a writer.

Unfortunately, this kind of outcome is not common. Misguided into feeling that they must resolve their sexual fantasies by boundary testing, many men feel under pressure to come up with a yes-or-no answer as to whether a woman will be sexually interested in them. The game-playing element becomes clear when we note how often the objective is simply that: to discover that a woman is indeed sexually available—to "score"—rather than to develop a rewarding relationship with her.

The masculine tendency to press for a resolution at the physical rather than the psychological level contributes to often-disastrous conflicts between men's and women's boundary and fantasy agendas—and to incidents of unwelcome sexual behavior that are now seen as sexually harassing. When a woman's fantasy creates a nonsexualized safety zone and the fantasized man exposes her to his sexuality by boundary testing, her fantasy can rapidly shift from perceiving the man as someone she admires to experiencing him as a monster who is tormenting her. A similar process occurs in men. When a woman who is the object of his sexual fantasy rebuffs a man's boundary advances, his fantasy can easily turn *her* into a monster, especially if she voices an official complaint about his behavior.

David Mamet's play *Oleanna* opens with a subtle boundary tension between a male professor and a female student who comes to one of his office hours. The student eventually brings a sexual harassment complaint against the professor. But by the play's end, Mamet has successfully turned both characters into monster caricatures. Performances of his drama were so darkly successful in stimulating the monsters within that there were many reports of couples screaming at each other in gender war as they left the theater.

Some real monsters do indeed exist: Both men and women can become destructive when there is gender conflict. But it is particularly tragic when a man or a woman who has made a mistake in his or her sexual-boundary behavior, but is willing to understand and correct that mistake, is identified as a monster. Most people *are* ready to draw upon their more reasonable selves and respond to current sexual harassment policies. For men, the central task is to find a more internalized, reflective way of resolving sexual fantasies, which includes learning to live with them for long periods of time without pushing for resolution on the physical level—to hew to boundary respecting. For women, increased reasonableness means not making monsters of men who, if they make a misstep, show a genuine capacity for learning new ways of managing their boundary behavior—and in some instances developing true empathy for the experience of women.

## HEALING MOMENTS

Healing moments don't occur very often when men and women get into boundary problems with each other. But as long as neither party has engaged in egregious behavior, I think that most people of goodwill, common decency, and some reasonableness should be able to wrest a satisfactory ending from a potential disaster. If they can't do it one-to-one, they should by all means call in someone who can mediate the process. Human resources officers at work and sexual harassment officers at schools are increasingly developing the skills to bring constructive endings to boundary misunderstandings and offenses that have the potential to lead to harassment charges.

Because I like healing moments, let me tell you what happened to Tom and Linda after their debacle, which left Linda feeling traumatized and defeated, and Tom walking around in a state of depression and anxiety, realizing he had done something terribly wrong. So shaken both were by the experience that they avoided each other at work for as long as they could. Linda began having uneasy dreams of men invading her house, instead of exhilarating reveries about the work she and Tom would do together. She would wake from these dreams in the middle of the night feeling that Tom was a dangerous man and resolve to file an official harassment complaint about him in the morning. But when morning came, she would go to work feeling too numb to do anything about what had happened, wishing she could sever the entire incident from her life.

Tom did not sleep easily either. He had a dream in which he was beckoned by a woman he found attractive. As he approached her, she sprouted claws and fangs, causing him to turn and flee, but he could not escape her grasp and awoke feeling her grip on him. At work, depressed and lifeless, he walked around afraid he would be fired, if not for sexual harassment then for incompetence. To distract himself, he tried working up an erotic fantasy about another woman at work, but it went nowhere.

Four days after the incident, Tom knocked on Linda's office door and asked if he could come in to discuss finalizing their project. Hesitantly she invited him in, simultaneously fearful and relieved to see him there. For several moments they sat silently side by side at her desk, looking at the memo and drawings. Then, before getting to work, Tom looked Linda steadily in the eye and said, "Linda, I'm really sorry about the other day. It won't happen again."

Linda held back her tears; she could hardly speak. "Thanks," she managed. "Can we go back to work now?" They started to attend to the project, then she found some more words. "Tom, when I touched you the other day, I was very excited about what we were doing, and I realized that you were unique in my life here. I didn't mean to lead you on. I don't like it that you took it sexually. I think we're good for each other creatively, but to me it has nothing to do with sex. Can you accept that?"

Tom, tense and sober until that moment, brightened up a bit. "Linda, I would do anything to have that moment I touched you back, but I can't. You're right—the chemistry between us got me thinking in a sexual direction, but I know it doesn't have to. There's enough going on between us in other ways. I hope you'll trust me enough sometime so that we can do good work together again."

It took Tom and Linda six more months to restore the creative flow and ease that had preceded their boundary problem. A year later, each dating someone else, they left InfoTech and together opened their own ad agency. Five years later, they run one of the most successful agencies in Silicon Valley, specializing in multimedia promotions for high-tech companies. Each has a family now, and they occasionally visit together. Tom does some pro bono work for a local women's crisis center. Linda feels that, against the odds, she has found a true professional sense of place, and she will still, very occasionally, touch a man's arm in conversation.

# 5. HOW HARASSMENT HAPPENS

*Sexual Coercion, Varieties of Boundary Crossings, and Gender Harassment*

Judy sits with Dave, her supervisor, looking over a report she has drafted on the performance of their Kansas City office. Dave, after uttering a series of indecipherable "um-hmms," suddenly grabs the report, gets up, and heads for the door. "Sorry, gotta go, Judy," he says on his way out. "I'll get back to you tomorrow about this, unless you're still here when I get back at five-thirty."

Judy is stunned. Dave has been growing more abrupt and arbitrary with her in the last two weeks. In the six months since her husband moved out, there has never been a problem about her clearly expressed and agreed-upon need to leave the office each day promptly at five to pick her two kids up at after-school day care. She leaves at her customary time but keeps processing the day's events and does not sleep well.

When Judy opens the office the next morning, the first thing she sees on her desk is the report she had left with Dave, covered with red markings. The phone rings. "Judy, this is Dave. I'm in the car heading over to Y-Tech. That document you gave me has serious problems. I need to talk to you about it when I get back to the office at six. If you're not there, I'll stop by your house tonight to go over it." The phone connection breaks. Judy wonders whether Dave wants her fired, wants her body, or wants both.

Dave does indeed show up at her house—at eight P.M. His appearance is clearly not welcome; on the doorstep, Judy says it's not a good time for her, and she smells alcohol on Dave's breath. But he makes a plea for the professional necessity of working on the report for just a little while, and Judy lets him in.

She asks Dave to have a seat at the kitchen table, excuses herself briefly to tuck her kids into bed, then comes downstairs. She finds Dave sprawled on the living-room sofa, the report next to him. A knot forms in Judy's stomach; her emotions tell her he is an unwanted intruder and to call the police. But her social management skills remind her that he is her boss. So she asks him to bring the report to the kitchen table. Dave waves it at her and says, "Why don't you come over here and sit next to me? I think we'll be able to work on the report after we get to know each other a little better."

Now Judy is certain of Dave's purpose, and an alarm goes off inside. She says, "Absolutely not. I don't want to get to know you better. But if you want to work on the report, bring it into the kitchen." Dave gets up, tosses the pages onto the coffee table, and heads for the door. "Take a look at it, and we'll discuss it in the morning," he tells her in an angry voice, and lets himself out of her house.

Now that we have explored the psychological and cultural underpinnings of sexual harassment, let's take a more systematic look at the scenarios through which it typically plays itself out in school and the workplace. Dave and Judy's story includes the most important elements of sexual harassment already discussed and adds significant new factors that are discussed below. Acting according to the sex-role spillover effect, Dave is managing his sexual boundaries and fantasies in the workplace just as men sometimes do in purely social situations.

Because a very clear line has now been drawn between the way people behave professionally and personally, we must subject our sexual boundary behavior to a very different standard at work and at school than we do in our private lives. But there is still disagreement about when a specific incident of unwelcome sexual behavior creates a hostile environment. If we are to have a better understanding of how *not* to harass, and to feel that we are on more solid ground should we want to complain about *being* harassed, this point urgently needs clarifying.

Toward that end, this chapter describes a classification for sexual-boundary behavior of minor, major, and egregious boundary crossings that should help us identify when the line that defines sexual harassment has been breached. Chapters 6 and 7, in turn, will build upon this classification and recommend a wide range of strategies for intervening in, and preventing, sexual harassment.

### HARASSMENT BETWEEN PEOPLE OF UNEQUAL POWER

Dave and Judy's case focuses on the particular problems of harassment between people of unequal authority. Dave is Judy's boss. When two people have unequal power and status at work or at school, we must judge the implications of sexual boundary behavior much more carefully than when they are co-workers. Although reporting any instance of possible sexual harassment is stressful, it is much easier for Winnie to go to the human resources department and discuss co-worker Ed's neck rubs than it will be for Judy to lodge a complaint about the behavior of a man who controls virtually every aspect of her job.

Ed and Winnie, like Tom and Linda, were equals on the organizational power chart. Another incident of harassment between equals—the sexually unwelcome notes and letters Kerry Ellison received—was the basis for the Reasonable Woman decision. Harassment between equals can be egregious and in its most severe form may culminate in everyone's worst nightmare: a spurned or discharged worker returning to work to exact revenge through violent assault. But the moment harassment involves two people of *unequal* status, the possibility for coercion and abuse of power is raised enormously. We see this clearly in Judy's and Dave's situation. As Judy instantly recognizes, Dave might want her body, her job, or both. When the person harassing is in a position to evaluate your work performance and make decisions about hiring and firing you, you have far more than your sexual boundaries to defend. Your failure to keep your superior "happy" with you may mean economic ruin or disastrously interrupt your career or academic path.

The psychological consequences of facing these possibilities are devastating. Company sexual harassment policies, backed up by law, are specifically designed to deter the kind of consequences that Judy fears from having rebuffed Dave, and to punish people who actually engage in such behavior. But an individual nonetheless faces a long and uphill road to legal, financial, and psychological recovery even from provable sexual harassment.

Given situations like Judy's, it is no mystery that only a small percentage of harassment episodes are ever reported. Typically, people who are harassed by those in authority try to manage the situation on their own, without putting their job at risk, rather than elevate the conflict to a harassment complaint.

For every harassed person whose complaint reaches an official forum—be it the company's own investigation resources, the EEOC, or a court of law—there are thousands who try to hang in there with their harassers and minimize the damage. A woman is in an appalling bind when taking action would mean threatening the career of the supervisor or teacher who determines everything from her day-to-day work conditions to her career path—and possibly the security of her entire family.

Although it is illegal for a supervisor to retaliate against people who have filed harassment complaints, the potential complainant is often very vulnerable. Judy, a single mother, depends on her job for both herself and her children. There are many subtle ways that Dave could retaliate against either her maintaining her boundaries that night or a decision to file an official complaint.

We still have a long way to go before the sexual boundary *behaviors* mandated by harassment law are reflected in sexual boundary *values*. While we can certainly continue to improve procedures that will encourage people to feel safer about reporting harassing incidents, they will be insufficient to fully protect most of those whose entire economic and psychological well-being can be instantly compromised when someone in authority harasses them.

## COERCIVE SEXUAL HARASSMENT

An element of coercion is always involved when someone of greater status within an organization behaves in a sexual way toward someone of lesser status. Sexual coercion can be hidden, or attempts may be made to deny it by redefining the context as "social" rather than work or school related. But consenting sexual behavior between adults requires freedom from all coercive factors, however subtle. There is no such freedom when the person who crosses the sexual boundaries has immediate or long-term power over the other person's working or learning conditions.

When Judy did not "consent" to take part in the sexual fantasy that lay behind Dave's visit to her home, he became angry. Given the coercion implicit in this situation, even if Judy had gone over to the couch and allowed Dave to touch her, her behavior would not have been truly "consenting." In fact, the very first sexual harassment case to reach the U.S. Supreme Court (*Meritor v. Vinson*, 1986) affirmed that there is a difference between true consent to engage in sex and apparent consent that is, in fact, coerced. *Meritor* stated the basis for this finding as follows: "Vinson's supervisor made repeated demands for sexual favors, usually at work, both during and after business hours. Vinson initially refused her employer's sexual advances, but eventually acceded because she feared losing her job. They had intercourse over forty times. . . . The [Supreme] Court had no difficulty finding this environment hostile." This statement was quoted in the Reasonable Woman decision five years later.

### Covert Quid Pro Quo Harassment

While quid pro quo harassment itself (jobs-for-sex, sex-for-jobs) constitutes a very small percentage of sexual harassment incidents, a covert quid pro quo threat is an element in sexual coercion. In the incident on Judy's sofa, since Dave did nothing that was definitively sexual and made no explicit demand for sex in exchange for her keeping her job, he might even argue that he had made a legitimate attempt at intimacy.

Should Judy come to work the next day and be fired, however, she would have a fairly good case that it had happened because she had refused to comply with Dave's agenda the previous evening. In fact, one reason that overt quid pro quo harassment is so infrequent is that it can so easily be

hidden. Suppose that, instead of firing her, Dave makes it extremely difficult for Judy to do her job over the next three or four weeks, and then fires
her for alleged work deficiencies. Should she decide to pursue sexual harassment charges against Dave, the basis for her case is unlikely to be quid
pro quo harassment; it would probably be a hostile work environment that
resulted from the way Dave behaved toward her in her home, which was
work related. But lurking in the background and at the heart of many of
these hostile environment cases *is* an implicit quid pro quo. Moreover,
because it coerces sex from someone in a weaker position, quid pro quo
harassment entails the possibility of rape.

In the notorious Tailhook incident, I believe Lieutenant Paula Coughlin's multimillion-dollar jury verdict stemmed from the jury's—and the
public's—distaste for sexual coercion. Although Coughlin was not literally
raped, being forced to run a gauntlet of sexually pawing Navy officers
strongly conveys the rape mentality that is in place in any degree of sexual
coercion.

## THE SEVERITY OF SEXUAL HARASSMENT:
## TYPES OF BOUNDARY CROSSINGS

Sexual boundaries between people are challenged, tested, and at times
crossed or violated in certain noticeable patterns. Learning to recognize
these patterns, and the degrees of severity of boundary crossings as they
typically arise in the workplace, can help us both to prevent harassing
behavior and to improve the way we deal with it when it occurs.

Boundary crossings can be classified as minor, major, and egregious. In
general, *minor* boundary crossings will not lead to harassment charges; *major*
ones are likely to lead to charges; and *egregious* ones, when verified, should
cause the harasser to be dismissed and place the organization at risk for
payment of damages. There are some exceptions to these outcomes, however, because legally the severity of the boundary crossing must be judged
in relation to other factors such as the degree of coercion, degree of
welcomeness, degree of previous notice, and degree of contribution to a
hostile working environment.

Because the boundary-crossing behavior itself is what sexual harassment
is about, it is important to define our terms. First, *boundary crossing* refers to

any behavior, verbal or nonverbal, that is sexual in nature or otherwise impacts on an individual's sense of privacy and personal space. *Verbal behavior* refers to comments made to, about, and around a person. Nonverbal behavior consists of touches, looks, and gestures, whether directed to an individual or going on around him or her; the delivery of sexually oriented visual or written material; or the posting of such material in a public place. Sexually oriented material posted in public places used to be confined to girlie calendars and posters on walls, or jokes and cartoons on bulletin boards. Today, with the prevalence of faxes, e-mail, and Internet and other on-line services, sexually oriented material that is not strictly private can be perceived as a boundary crossing of a minor, major, or egregious nature.

It is essential to remember that the severity of a boundary crossing is primarily judged by the person whose boundaries are being impacted by the behavior. In other words, it is *the recipient's own experience* of the behavior that determines its severity. This doesn't mean that a person can single-handedly decide that he or she was harassed—there are also checks and balances against making an individual's subjective opinion the sole measurement of harassment. A unanimous Supreme Court in 1993 set the latest standard for sexual harassment in *Harris v. Forklift Systems:* It is unwelcome sexual behavior that a Reasonable Person in the same circumstances would find sufficient to create a hostile working environment. (Although the Court did not use the term *Reasonable Woman* here, a Reasonable Person is implicitly either a Reasonable Woman or a Reasonable Man, depending on who is bringing the harassment charge.) With this decision, the Court reaffirmed its focus on the experience and judgment of the person whose boundaries have been crossed.

### Minor Boundary Crossings

Boundary crossings can be minor if the recipient did not experience the behavior as sexual or offensive. If someone brushes against your body at work, it is a boundary crossing, but if you are sure that it was inadvertent and without sexual intent, it is a minor boundary crossing.

Even if someone brushes against your intimate parts, it may be accidental or harmless and nothing to take particular note of. On the other hand, if this behavior is repeated a few times, it might go from a minor to a major sexually harassing boundary crossing fairly quickly.

It's also a minor boundary crossing if someone pats you encouragingly on the shoulder, comments on your appearance, or asks you to lunch or dinner in a way that you find nonsexual, nonoffensive, and noncoercive. Even if you realize in thinking about it afterward that the other person was expressing some sexual interest, it remains a minor boundary event if you have had no problem with it and feel that your response was respected.

Sometimes one individual will consider minor what many others would classify as a major or even an egregious boundary crossing. A woman who worked at a video store was being interviewed by a sexual harassment researcher about comments and touches she had received from customers. She reported that an elderly man who was a regular customer had once put his hand on her buttocks when she was bending down to reshelve a tape, telling her, "Better watch where you point that, honey." When asked how she felt about this, she told the researcher, "Oh, that's just George. He's harmless." Another woman in the same situation, or the same woman being touched by a younger man whose requests for dates she may have rejected, might experience this kind of touch and comment as clearly harassing.

The subjective nature of judging boundary crossings cuts both ways. Some people do not take offense at certain behaviors, allowing for a little "harmless" sexual conversation. Others do not take well to even a very mild, innocently intended sexual comment. Either way, the point is that the experience and dignity of the recipient of the behavior are central considerations in judging any boundary crossing.

### Turning a Minor Boundary Crossing into a Major One

Whether a boundary-crossing event remains minor depends to a great extent on whether the behavior is repeated and how the response to it is handled.

> Helen works as a paralegal for a large law firm. One afternoon a partner comes up behind her in the library as she is looking for a book, reaches high above her for a book of his own, and in the process leans against her from the rear, excusing himself with a quick "sorry" before giving her a sheepish look and scurrying away. Because he has never engaged in any previous untoward

behavior, Helen is willing to let the incident go. Although it felt intentional to her, she allows for the possibility that the bodily contact was truly accidental, with no sexual intent—as if, in effect, she were a piece of furniture in the way of his reach.

All goes well for another six weeks; then virtually the same thing happens. This time, just as the attorney gets his book and turns again for a quick apology, another partner enters the library. Seething with anger and about to read the man the riot act, Helen instead gives him a withering, angry look that his colleague cannot see.

Five years later, this partner has never come physically near her again and continues to treat her in a professional though somewhat distant way whenever their paths cross.

Helen's withering look in that one second put the man "on notice" more effectively than many angry words might have. Clearly he had pushed his luck and made a minor boundary crossing into a major one, but he was spared an official harassment complaint only because he took the notice seriously.

In truth, most people in the workplace would rather view a one-time boundary event—such as a touch, a comment, or a request for a date—as a minor, nonharassing crossing, as Helen did the first time, if there is any ambiguity at all about it. It takes not "getting it" and repeating the behavior to turn it into a major event.

But the usual way many people deal with a one-time event—by sloughing it off—is itself a problem. If you don't make something of a deal about the incident—if you basically ignore it—you do not give the person who acted inappropriately explicit notice that what he did was unwelcome. Without such a signal, feedback-loop skills may not come into play; the offender may well need such feedback.

A valid way to give notice at this level is to express it nonverbally, as Helen did. For legal purposes, it is often considered notice to walk away from a situation in which another person is getting too close physically, or to leave an area where sexualized joking and bantering are occurring.

Often this kind of notice is preferable to a woman stopping everything and saying, "Gil, I'm not going to make a big deal of what just happened because maybe you really didn't mean to brush my breast, but just don't ever do it again." In fact, by articulating what has happened in this way, she makes the incident into a reasonably big deal. This can be very effective. But for people who do not want to be this explicit, nonverbal signaling is acceptable. Whatever notice is given, the person whose boundaries have been crossed must feel thereafter that her rights and wishes are being respected. If she signals or actually asks that a certain kind of touching or sexual comment not be repeated, and that is the end of it, she knows she is being allowed to set boundaries for herself that she feels are proper. Even if she felt some degree of disrespect in the initial boundary crossing, respect is restored when her response has a positive effect on the behavior of those around her.

### Protecting Fantasies

Unfortunately, even when a woman serves mild notice, a troublesome psychological pattern can lead to behavior opposite to what she wants. Jerilyn, a woman in her late twenties who had just started work as a claims examiner for a medical insurance company, asked a male co-worker who had approached her a bit too closely at the copy machine to please be more careful. While he seemed to take the matter well, Jerilyn later discovered that another man in the office who had learned about the incident had since been referring to her as "Ms. Sensi-buns," and several other men in the office were having fun with this name.

Calling a worker by a derogatory nickname, especially one with a sexual connotation, is a major boundary crossing. This minor boundary crossing, which need have gone no further, became a major one, with outside people involved. We can credit our old friend sex-role spillover behavior with effecting the transformation. A not-uncommon masculine response to a woman who tries to control her own sexual boundaries is to attempt to discredit, humiliate, or scapegoat her, even when her reaction has been mild. It is easy to see how much more intense this type of male response can become if she lodges an official complaint or actually files a lawsuit.

Men respond this way in an effort to protect their sexual fantasies. Some men walk around with a free-floating fantasy that all women they encounter are potentially sexually available. When a woman's behavior discourages this fantasy, the man tries to discredit, deny, or reinterpret it. Some researchers advance a theory, which I find credible, that there is a sociobiological source for this kind of behavior left over from a time when the survival of the species depended on males checking out all females they encountered for possible propagation. (Indeed, we can also see the traces of this impulse in Level B masculine boundary testing.) But whether or not this theory is valid, it does not excuse such repugnant behavior.

## Persistent Requests: Does No Mean Yes?

Even simple workplace requests for dates are minor boundary crossings. A date is any one-to-one meeting that is not an ordinary part of working together. This includes having lunch, coffee, tea, a drink, or dinner together, as well as evening and weekend meetings. Even if a man does it graciously, masking all Level B fantasizing, asking someone he works with for a date is a boundary-crossing event because it is a request for greater intimacy.

Requests for dates, and even dates themselves, are not at all uncommon. Why is it, then, that a great many cases of workplace harassment begin with such requests? The one-word answer is *persistence*. Persisting after a simple no is another sure way to turn a minor boundary crossing into a major one. Indeed, this could be a rule for many boundary-crossing acts: once is minor; twice, after notice of unwelcomeness is given, is major; three or four times move it toward egregiousness.

Persistence is another form of "protecting the fantasy," akin to belittling and scapegoating women who don't play their desired parts in men's fantasies. Why are men so prone to persist when women say no? Simply put, because the woman in their fantasies is saying yes, and they prefer yes to no. The "When she says no, it means yes" mindset is also explainable in terms of protecting the fantasy. So is its variant: "Her words said no, but her body [eyes, clothes, stance] said yes." The problem is not the fantasy itself; it is the effort to impose it on another.

## Major Boundary Crossings

Are major boundary crossings, then, nothing other than minor boundary crossings that have escalated because someone didn't take seriously a message to cease and desist? In general, yes. The hallmark of a major boundary crossing is that it is unmistakably sexual in nature. As we have seen, minor boundary crossings leave room for uncertainty about whether the incident was sexual, and the person experiencing the behavior is usually willing to extend the benefit of the doubt to the other, at least for one time. Many physical hoverings and seemingly accidental touches fall into this category. But regardless of whether it is repeated, a physical or verbal act that is clearly sexual is a major boundary crossing.

Who is the judge of whether an act is unmistakably sexual? Again, it is the person who experiences the behavior, with the customary caveat that a reasonable person in the same circumstances could experience it similarly. If every time Joe gets up to go to the water cooler, Jill thinks he is coming on to her, even though he does not pass her desk, look at, or even address her, her judgment is most likely *un*reasonable. But if it turns out that he has continually been leaving her notes saying, "When I go to the water cooler, I want you to meet me there," then it is entirely reasonable for her to feel that he is sending her a sexual message and that his behavior is a major boundary crossing.

When a man tells a woman at work, "You're looking good today," it may be minor; there is room for uncertainty about whether his intent is sexual, some of which can be determined by his tone, accompanying looks, body language, and any history of making comments like this in the past. But when standing too close, leering, staring at body parts, or brushing against someone cannot reasonably be understood as inadvertent, then it is a major boundary crossing. And when a man says, "You sure fill out that sweater," his comment is unmistakably sexual and a major boundary crossing.

Asking a woman to lunch, dinner, or even for a drink can be unwelcome behavior even if it's done nicely, yet the request can remain a minor boundary crossing. But it is unmistakably sexual to say to a woman at work, "I bet you'd like some of the tapes I have at home—why don't you come watch them with me?" or "I see you've been working on your tan—I know this great little beach I can take you where you can lose those tan lines."

## It's a Boundary Crossing, But Is It Harassment?

As offensive as many of these major boundary crossings sound, neither minor nor major ones in themselves constitute sexual harassment. In order to be judged as sexually harassing, the boundary crossing typically also has to (1) be unwelcome, (2) be repeated after the person engaging in the behavior has been put on notice that it is unwelcome, and (3) demonstrably create a hostile working environment, as judged by a reasonable person in the same circumstances.

As we have seen, coercion is a factor in determining whether a working environment is hostile. The degree of coercion may be difficult to assess when the individuals concerned are peers, although it is unambiguous if physical force is involved or suggested. A woman who is lured to an isolated area in the workplace where she cannot fend off forcible physical advances is not only in a coercive situation but in one that may qualify as criminal sexual assault or rape. However, when a person of greater authority crosses the boundaries of someone of lesser authority, coercion is a critical determinant of hostility in the working environment. In situations where inequality of status does not allow for coercion-free behavior, even what would otherwise be a minor boundary crossing—say, a one-time request for a date—can become a major boundary event and, unless the other person welcomes it, be perceived as coercive and innately harassing.

When a CEO asks a younger, newly hired secretary for a date, even if she says yes, he is putting himself at risk for harassing should she complain some time in the future that she felt coerced when he invited her. Although it may be hard to determine whether coercion exists when somebody says yes, common sense and a "reasonable" understanding of the experience of people in positions of lesser power allow us to recognize when a boundary crossing involves coercion.

A determination of sexual harassment that meets certain criteria has to be made only if a formal complaint has been filed and the company, the EEOC, a state agency, or a court needs to arrive at an official ruling of whether the behavior is sexually harassing. Most issues of workplace harassment are dealt with on a less formal basis, by human resources and other personnel, as part of a day-to-day effort to reduce misunderstanding and enhance mutual respect among workers. These discussions of the nuances of boundary crossings are intended not to suggest that people should offer legal opinions about the behavior in question but to focus awareness on the meaning and impact of boundary behaviors so that everyone in the workplace has an opportunity to act with fuller knowledge of what is involved.

### "I'll Just Drop By Your House"

Stories of sexual harassment disasters that began with someone "just drop-ping by" someone else's house are legion. This situation is such a setup for sexual fantasies to go out of control that "just dropping by" constitutes a category in itself of major boundary crossing.

Sexual harassment cases are replete with workers "dropping by" or get-ting others to come over to their home. In the Reasonable Woman case, the man who wrote Kerry Ellison those unwelcome admiring notes had originally taken her to lunch at a restaurant near the IRS headquarters where they worked. After lunch, to which he drove her in his car, he told her he had to swing by his home to pick up his son's forgotten school lunch. She accompanied him inside, where, as Judge Beezer noted, "he gave Ellison a tour of his house."

At this level of workplace acquaintanceship, before anything strange or patently unwelcome has occurred, it is difficult to object to an errand suggesting that a co-worker is a devoted family man. Still, while such maneuvers may be completely innocent, they are more likely to be classic exercises in Level A versus Level B communication. At Level A "dropping by" someone's home has a completely legitimate ostensible purpose; at level B, it is a *major* boundary crossing into intimate space, and the person setting it up (usually a man) may be looking very closely for clues that the other person (usually a woman) is responding to the sexual boundary-testing message. If a woman so much as accepts a glass of wine during a drop-by-home incident, she may be unintentionally signaling, at least in the language the man has traditionally learned, that she now regards this as a social rather than a professional situation. If it were in fact a social visit, then *workplace* sexual harassment standards would not apply. But if there is *any* work connection at all, the harassment standards do apply, no matter how strong the wish to ignore them.

A work connection, not a social visit, was the excuse for the visit Dave made to Judy's house at eight that evening, and it was a major boundary crossing. But Judy was well aware that his motive for "stopping by" might be unrelated to work, and she viewed his visit as unwelcome. Their unequal status added a coercive element to what was already a major boundary crossing. But regardless of status, unless a woman explicitly welcomes a visit as purely social, every incident of dropping by home should be seen not only as a major boundary crossing but as an opportunity for significant sexual boundary testing to occur.

## Hotel Rooms, Isolation, and Creating Fantasy Space

"Just dropping by" is a potentially dangerous type of major boundary crossing, bordering on the egregious. What is going on is an attempt to get a co-worker into physical circumstances that are associated with private, intimate behavior rather than with work. The home is not the only such circumstance. Workplaces usually have remote storerooms or other un-populated areas. Sometimes these places are notorious trysting grounds—or exist as such in some people's fantasies.

It is usually not harassment if two co-workers, of absolutely equal status, who both welcome it with no trace of coercion, want to sneak off and be sexual together. But as previously described, it is a different matter entirely if a woman finds herself in a solitary place where she cannot fight off unwanted physical advances. Coercion clearly exists under such circum-stances, whether the two individuals are peers or one is the other's superior.

Other circumstances where people may try to become intimate with co-workers are cocktail lounges, cars, restaurants, or hotel rooms while on the road. In general, a dinner date after hours is light-years away from a lunch date during working hours. (A true *working* dinner between co-workers, whether locally or on the road, is a different matter; this is not a date, which is a social event.) The key factor is an attempt to isolate someone from the peer-group community of the usual working environment. Like just-dropping-bys, or journeys to a remote room in the workplace, these major boundary crossings are potentially dangerous instances of the power-ful influence of some men's sexual fantasy life on their behavior.

## Egregious Boundary Crossings

Egregious boundary crossings are words and actions so clearly offensive that there can be no serious debate about whether they are acts of sexual harassment. When a man puts M&M's in a woman's breast pocket, as in the Baker & MacKenzie case, it might be a minor boundary crossing if he carefully dropped them into her pocket without touching her—although that is virtually a physical impossibility—and she was amused by it. It is a major boundary violation if he so much as brushes her clothing with his hand. But when he allows his hand to linger even a moment to touch her breast, it is an egregious boundary violation. This kind of sex-role spillover behavior is known, universally, as "copping a feel."

"Copping a feel," when someone intentionally makes contact with someone else's breast, buttock, or genital area without permission or notice that it is welcome, is one of the more recognizable forms of egregious boundary crossing. "I couldn't believe it," fifty-two-year-old Hannah told me. "I've been Mr. Wade's administrative assistant for two years. He's been a little flirtatious, but he never crossed any lines that I couldn't just ignore. The other day he just comes up to me, cups my breast in his hand, and says, 'You're gaining a little weight, Hannah. Looks nice!' I was so completely stunned, I couldn't say anything. Then I went to the bathroom and threw up."

One would like to think that halfway through the 1990s, after the widespread publicity about sexual harassment, this kind of behavior would have all but disappeared. It hasn't, and reports about such egregious boundary crossings surface all the time. Just reaching out and touching someone is still deeply programmed into the sex-role behavior of men. For instance, the Senate Ethics Committee resolution for the investigation of Senator Packwood, which culminated in its unanimous vote in September 1995 to expel him, detailed alleged incidents of unwanted sexual touching by the senator toward sixteen different women between 1969 and 1990. Five of the allegations describe him "forcing his tongue" into a woman's mouth, and many others describe forceful, unwanted touching, such as an incident in which he "grabbed the staff assistant, pinned her against a wall or desk, held her hair with one hand . . . fondling her with his other hand and kissed her."

In general, egregious boundary crossings are not at all subtle; they are acts of sexual imposition that can run well beyond offensive words and acts to sexual assault, intimidation, and rape. A man may begin by "copping a feel" but move on to more forceful touching, blocking a doorway, or verbally threatening harm if a woman doesn't comply sexually. Although this is still sexual harassment, we have entered the realm of possible criminal behavior as well.

In fact, a shocking number of harassing acts, especially egregious boundary crossings, are potentially criminal acts. If a man walks up to a woman on the street and snaps her underwear, we will immediately consider calling the police. Yet the same behavior between a man and his secretary has been an often-accepted boundary-testing ritual, as if he has certain rights over her body because she agreed to take the job.

Clearly, all quid pro quo invitations are inherently egregious boundary crossings. Telling someone she must engage in sexual behavior in order to get, keep, or receive some privilege on the job is an outright act of sexual coercion. Simply suggesting to someone as a job-advancing tactic that she *consider* a sexual act is an equally intimidating act of quid pro quo harassment. A woman I once interviewed told me that she went to her boss for her ninety-day performance evaluation, which was to change her job status from probationary to permanent. Her boss promptly unbuckled his belt, zipped down his fly, and said, "Okay, I'm going to evaluate your performance." He did not persist when she got up and walked out of the office. But because she could not afford to quit the job immediately, she came to work terrorized from that day on.

Outright quid pro quo harassment like this is uncommon, as we have noted, but any boundary crossing becomes egregious if it holds the implication of power. When Dave "dropped by" Judy's house, his boundary crossing was egregious because he used his coercive power as her boss to force himself past her doorstep, even after she told him it was not a good time for his visit. If a flirtatious co-worker drops by but, when told not to come in, promptly departs without threat or undue persistence, the incident does qualify as a major boundary crossing because it enters intimate space—but it is not egregious unless physical or psychologically coercive power is wielded.

### "But I Can Get Away With It"

When a man engages in egregious boundary crossing, somewhere inside him is the fantasy that the woman he touches will actually *enjoy* it. An additional fantasy that usually accompanies boundary-crossing behavior is that "I can get away with it." Jim, a forty-two-year-old formerly up-and-coming executive, was sent to me for consultation by his company after coming up behind his new secretary and snapping the waistband of her underwear. He was frank about what he had done:

I've done stuff like that fifty times. We get a lot of temps in and out of the office, and I kind of like to test them that way—they usually just laugh it off and move away. I even ended up sleeping with one of them. I guess I got lulled into thinking I could just do it. My word against theirs, you know. In fact, I just denied it when I was finally called on it by this woman. Still would have gotten away with it, but it was my bad luck that they found two others who said I did the same thing to them. I guess it's time to change my ways.

Jim's way of looking at this incident contains other lessons about sexual harassment. The fact that one secretary slept with him is a major fantasy reinforcer. That's the way this kind of fantasy thinking works: The mind-set calculates odds and risks irrationally. One payoff out of fifty egregious boundary crossings may be enough to keep alive the fantasy that the next woman will enjoy it.

Every workplace now bears a clear responsibility to intervene in the part of the fantasy that says "I can get away with it." As workplace norms evolve toward making harassment unacceptable, fewer men will risk egregious and other boundary crossings under the illusion that they can get away with it. They may not abandon the deeper level of the fantasy that believes that a woman they hardly know will respond to them sexually. But today we are drawing fresh boundaries by sending out the new message that men no longer have the ancient license to test out their fantasies with impunity.

## GENDER HARASSMENT

Gender harassment is a very different animal from sexual harassment. While I believe that much harassment is sexually motivated boundary behavior gone terribly wrong, gender harassment is rooted in sheer hatred of people who are different from oneself and in attempts to exert power over them. We know a great deal about prejudice and bigotry on the basis of otherness: those who are suspicious of or dislike an individual or a group because it differs from us in religion, race, skin color, ethnicity, sexual orientation, nationality, social class—the list is endless. In gender harassment the suspicion, dislike, or hatred is based on the person's gender. "He's just a prick like all the others." "I don't want to see another fucking cunt on this job."

The core of gender harassment is not sexual fantasy gone out of control; it is the denial of a person's essential humanness—justifying violence and, in its most extreme form, even killing. Gender harassment is played out through systematic efforts to keep the other gender (in our world, that almost always means women) out of the workplace. According to Louise Fitzgerald, a social psychologist and leading researcher on this problem, gender harassment is a workplace spillover of violence against women in our society, which includes domestic violence, battering, and rape. As such, it should be viewed as a raw assertion of power.

Fitzgerald's view is supported by the story that Kara, a woman I interviewed, told me. Although she had been hired as a highly skilled carpenter for a major building project, the contractor had her spend the first four months patrolling the grounds and picking up garbage. When she questioned this, the foreman told her, "Do you want the job or not?" He then muttered, barely under his breath, "Stupid bitch."

When Kara finally got to work on the building, she found that plywood catwalks near her were sometimes not secured, and that nail guns were being used in what she considered a careless manner. With stray nails whizzing near her like bullets, Kara realized that her life was in danger. Still, some of the men accepted her and were supportive, so she decided to tough it out and stay on the job, becoming extremely vigilant about where she stepped and what was going on around her. In fact, Kara said, she found she was beginning to miss the old days, when she was first breaking into the trade, when she merely got whistles, calls of "Hey, baby," offers of massage, and blunt invitations to perform specific sexual acts on her co-workers.

These sexual boundary violations turned into gender hatred and threats to Kara's life because her skills had developed to the point that some men now feared she was the first of a whole new class of people, women, with whom they would now have to compete for jobs. "We're going to be replaced by a goddamned cunt corps," as one man had bluntly put it.

One day a brick came flying off the building and hit Kara in the shoulder, breaking her collarbone. Although she could have returned to work when it healed, she decided that it was clearly too dangerous for her

on this job. Eventually she brought a sex-discrimination and sexual harassment lawsuit against the contractor, who vigorously defended his company's actions on the basis that everything she had experienced—the
garbage patrol, the job hazards, the loose plywood, even the falling brick—
were risks for everyone on the job, men and women alike. Thus, according
to the contractor, there had been no sex discrimination.

When her lawsuit came to trial, Kara's prospects seemed grim; it appeared that the contractor's arguments were going to prevail. But one of the
men who had befriended her on the job finally came forward, risking his
own position, to testify to the number of times that he heard the foreman
refer to her as "that goddam cunt." When the jury heard this, the contractor's house of cards fell. The defense quickly settled the case before the
jury reached a verdict.

Pure gender harassment is most likely to occur in work forces that have
been traditionally purely male. There is reason to hope that events like this
are chiefly the result of a painful period of transition, which will diminish
as more and more women enter the work force in a wider variety of
occupations, establishing new norms for expectations and behavior. It is
extremely difficult to fight deep-seated fears and prejudices. But at least we
now have a clearly stated ideal from which to draw. Equality is good for the
psyche, and for society.

# 6. A GUIDE FOR MEN

*Preventing Sexual Harassment and Responding*
*to a Complaint*

From speaking to hundreds of men in the last few years, it is evident to me that a revolutionary change in men's thinking about sexual harassment has already occurred. True, their boundary behavior is not always a model of restraint and propriety, and certainly no revolution has occurred in their private sexual fantasies. But there seems no question that men now realize that their sexual boundary behavior is, as never before, being *watched.* It is a radically new perception.

Some men accept this change and have become willing and interested participants in the momentous transformations taking place in sexual ethics. Others keep trying to laugh these changes off, hoping that the focus on sexual harassment will somehow magically go away. And many others, not surprisingly, are angry, defensive, and fearful. Even those who might want to live up to the new standards sometimes find themselves disoriented and resentful. But what is universal for all of them, whatever their feelings, is that they are now on the alert, knowing that their sexual boundary behavior is being held up to unprecedented scrutiny.

No one should underestimate the importance of this change in awareness, because as long as society could not even put a name to sexual harassment, it was impossible to identify it, much less to ask people to stop.

Under those circumstances it could be difficult for men to know when they had treated women in ways that were not respectful of their sexual boundaries. Women too lacked the vocabulary—and societal support—to express just what they found unwelcome and offensive. When behavior is "normal," it is so much a part of everyday life that it is invisible. Twenty years ago, scarcely an eyebrow would have been raised if a man ogled a woman in the workplace and said something like, "Oooo, baby, I like what I see!" Today, an "Oooo, baby" comment is considered a major boundary crossing because its sexual meaning is clear. If repeated even once after notice of its unwelcomeness has been served, the man saying it is likely to be subjected to severe sanctions. For the law now mandates that almost every educational setting and workplace comply with the EEOC sexual harassment guidelines.

## MEN ON THE ALERT: TURNING FEAR INTO CONSCIOUSNESS

What I see in men's fear, anxiety, anger, and edgy jokes is a heightened sensitivity to the new sexual boundaries. Even when they express this sensitivity defensively in an apparently "negative" form, there is no reason why it cannot be part of the dialogue about sexual harassment. This chapter suggests ways in which such feelings can be constructively addressed.

Take, for example, the case of Frank, whom I met in the elevator of my office building one day when he was working on a crew remodeling one of the suites. As the elevator door was closing on the ground floor, a woman in the lobby pushed the button to stop the door, looked inside the crowded elevator, and said, "I'll take the next one." When the door closed, Frank said, "Oh, baby, you should have gotten in here and squeezed in next to me!" In the silence that ensued, he looked around at the three other men and two women in the elevator. Addressing one of the men, he said, "Oops, I can't say that anymore—sexual harassment!"

Later that day, I went to the suite where Frank was working, introduced myself, and told him I was doing research on sexual harassment. I asked if he could spare a few minutes to talk to me about what had happened that morning. Frank, who was forty-five years old and divorced, warmed to the task:

> She was a good-looking babe, wasn't she? You were there, you saw! I'll bet every guy on the elevator wished he could have gotten close to her, including you, Doc. But I'm lucky that door closed and she didn't hear me say what I did. It could have been my job. Hell, it still could be my job if one of those ladies in

the elevator complains about me. Look, I like women—and I always treat them with respect, one on one. Saying stuff like that—it's just second nature. Just a way of making contact, you know? I'm harmless—I'd never do something to a lady she didn't want.

Yeah, I know, I turned it into a joke. But that's because I'm scared. We're all paranoid now. A woman so much as suggests you harassed her, and you're in big trouble. Almost doesn't matter anymore if you did it or not. I know they've had it bad over the years, but the balance has really swung the other way, and now we're the ones who are up against it.

A few days later, I was at a parents' meeting at the school my children attend, talking about the same subject to a man named George. George had graduated from a prestigious university and is a partner at an investment banking firm. He also teaches part-time in an MBA program. This is what he had to tell me:

This harassment thing is on our minds all the time, whenever there are women around us. You know, I'm *glad* there are more women in my profession—I've always supported them. But everybody's really scared. One misstep, and your career's over. And it's so subjective about what's harassing that you could get nailed just because you put your hand on a woman's shoulder going out the door. They want equality? Well, I also put my arm around men's shoulders going through doorways—to me it's part of the social graces I was raised with. Not that anyone's complained about me yet—but you get kind of jumpy thinking about it every time a woman comes near you.

Obviously Frank and George are saying much the same thing—and if you took your own survey, you'd find thoughts like these echoed by men everywhere. I consider Frank and George to be decent men. No, they're not perfect. Both are alert to issues of sexual harassment, sensitive to the fact that there are new and changing boundaries, respectful of women in their own eyes, and seemingly willing to learn what is required of them. Their anxieties and questions about sexual harassment are legitimate and must be addressed if there is going to be a cooperative rather than an antagonistic future for men and women working and learning together as equals.

Keeping in mind Frank, George, and all other men who wish to work in a peaceable way on the sexual harassment problem, I propose the following preventive steps to minimize the chances of a man's becoming embroiled in a sexual harassment complaint:

1. Identify your sexual fantasies, know when they are operating, and respect their power.
2. Acknowledge that fantasies are an unreliable guide to sexual boundary behavior.
3. While sexual fantasies are points of access to your inner life, keep them private unless you are sure they are welcome.
4. Take care of yourself physically and psychologically, and look for signs of depression.
5. All boundaries are two-person negotiations; hone the feedback loop to recognize what is unwelcome.

### I. Identify Your Sexual Fantasies

Sexual fantasies are extremely powerful experiences. They suddenly bring together many different parts of ourselves that usually function separately: Our biological and physical selves are acting in combination with our hopes, wishes, and even past wounds. As enacted or experienced in sexual fantasies, these feelings embody the range of our quests, both dark and light: for power, revenge, and hate, and for love, intimacy, and beauty. At the heart of our sexual fantasizing lies our attempt to enter the current of life itself—whether through physical procreation or through the creative experience of feeling more alive within.

Bob, a twenty-eight-year-old man who worked in an auto plant, was referred to me for a mild depression following a breakup with his girlfriend. Although he had no trouble going to his job, he told me that when he came home to his empty apartment, he felt half dead, as if his whole life had departed with his girlfriend. He painted a very bleak picture. Then his face suddenly took on a sly look. "It's weird, though," he said. "Last night this checkout girl at the supermarket gave me a special smile, and I walked out of there with a spring in my step, fantasizing about her. It didn't last that long, and it doesn't take away the pain, but whenever I think about her and that smile, I feel alive again. I feel like there's hope that I'll be over this."

Although I had previously considered that Bob might need antidepressant medication, I decided to hold off recommending it. Sure enough, over the next few weeks he completed his grieving and came back to life. He never saw the checkout girl again. But it was as if his image of her smile, and the sexual fantasizing that went along with it, were his own mental picture of his emerging, healing self.

### 2. Acknowledge that Fantasies Are an Unreliable Guide

Sexual fantasies are notoriously unreliable guides to what is actually going on in our interactions with others. The more powerful the fantasy, the more unrealistic is the information it generates about the interpersonal realm.

In some ways, men have it backward. They tend to overuse their fantasies in the very activity for which these are least valuable: judging the reality of what is going on with the women to whom they are attracted. In doing so, they fail to use the fantasies for what they are exceedingly good at: telling them more about *themselves*. A fantasy is an access point, a listening post as it were, to our fundamental psychobiological makeup. Sexual fantasies are too important to misuse as the basis for making social judgments.

An important first step is for a man simply to admit to himself that he does fantasize, and to notice all the places where sexual fantasy enters into his daily life.

His next step is to do his best to relinquish sexual fantasy as any sort of guide as to how he should behave toward other people. Men need to discover an entirely new orientation toward boundary behavior—a true two-person negotiation in which each person has veto power over unwelcome boundary behavior by the other. This negotiation is simply a conversation in which each listens to, attempts to understand, and then respects the other's wishes and needs.

Sometimes conversations of this sort can lead to a personal relationship in which each person *wants* to participate in the intimate world of the other, including his or her sexual fantasies. But the development of such intimacy is an unusual event, one to be savored. You cannot approach

others with any sort of expectation that they will be interested in participating in your fantasy life.

### 3. Keep Your Sexual Fantasies Private

It is important to work to conceal our sexual fantasies. A funny thing can
easily happen with fantasies: You think, "Uh-oh, I'll bet she knows what
I'm thinking," and a tinge of guilt, shame, and intrigue accompanies that
thought. But it's almost certainly wrong. She *doesn't* know what you're
thinking. Men project that women know these things because they wish it
were so; men have also become used to letting women play the role of
telling them what their feelings are. In fact, one of the most important
tasks in boundary management is to make very sure a woman *doesn't* know
what you're thinking by refusing to subject her to boundary-testing behavior. You can monitor the boundaries all you want, but it is essential to
cease testing out your fantasies.

Graham, a divorced man in his mid-thirties, had taken a shine to Jane, a
woman who worked in the cubicle across from his in a health insurance
claims office. Although they often had lunch together and chatted about
the daily office routine, Jane had never divulged any personal information.
Graham felt it would be out of line for him to try crossing over her
boundary, even with mild inquiries. After eight months his patience was
rewarded when Jane asked him if he'd like to have supper after work. Then
they began dating. Graham later told me that the first thing Jane said at
their dinner was, "I've never dated a man from work before; it always
seemed like it would be big trouble. But somehow I trust you, because even
with all our conversations, you've always respected my privacy."

Given that men's sexual fantasies come true only rarely, men must still
deal with all their energy. But how? One answer is that it's fine to continue
doing everything you are already doing to manage your sexual fantasies *in
private,* including masturbation, as long as your behavior is not harmful to
yourself or others.

Another way to channel the energy of fantasies is to seek their internal
meaning. There are many ways to do this: draw, paint, write, sing, keep a
diary, dream, share them with other men, perhaps even talk to a woman
you can trust who really wants to hear about your fantasies. Above all,
watch your boundaries carefully and keep the fantasies private. If you do

talk about them with someone at work, make sure it's out of range of anyone else, and don't let written or visual material from your fantasy life become accessible to others.

The Internet and other new on-line services are remarkably rich media for communication with others, as well as for playing out fantasy lives. But these networks pose the same difficult boundary questions that we are trying to work out elsewhere in our society. People have already been disciplined for sexual harassment, and for actual criminal behavior, resulting from crossing boundaries on-line. Those who want to connect at the fantasy level run into trouble because there is very little private space on-line. We have few guarantees that even personal e-mail will remain confidential. Anyone who posts a message in a forum, discussion group, chat room, Listserv, or Usenet news group has entered public space and will be held accountable to its standards.

### 4. Take Care of Yourself Physically and Psychologically

Another way to cope with sexual fantasies effectively is to keep yourself in reasonably healthy physical and psychological condition—and to have some fun. There are thousands of ways that men already do this; to each his own. Good physical exercise is a fundamental need. Some contact with nature and the outdoors can be valuable. Men's gatherings have become important in some circles. (Drumming and contacting the inner wild man are optional.) My favorite men's gathering is the truly ancient ritual of alternately sitting and standing with forty thousand others in a large structure and screaming my head off at people running around on a field with a ball—either a small round white one or a larger, brownish oblong one with pointy ends.

As for direct ways of working on psychological health, psychotherapy has a great deal to offer men at certain times of their lives. There are numerous kinds of therapy, and even some new medications, that can be extremely health promoting, if not life saving, at the right time.

Men who work extremely hard are notoriously poor at attending to their basic well-being. They become physically and psychologically run down, which can put them at risk for using poor judgment in making decisions about how to handle their fantasies and their boundaries. Some may live for years with untreated chronic depression. Instead of or in addition to medication, men have the option of psychotherapy to deal with depression and other psychological symptoms. My own school of therapy, the Jungian, has a special interest in helping people integrate into their daily lives the vast unconscious inner resources suggested by their dream and fantasy worlds; but I believe that the competence, integrity, and wisdom of the healer or therapist you work with, of any school, are far more important than are his or her underlying theoretical beliefs. Religious, spiritual, and meditative traditions also offer ways to cultivate inner life, healthy boundaries, values of non-harm, and wisdom. I recommend any that call to you.

Although depression has psychological ramifications, it is coming to be seen more and more as a biologically based condition, much like a hormonal or metabolic imbalance. Any man who feels as if he's living in shades of gray, with the happy moments either hard to find or impossible to respond to, should consult with a primary care physician or a psychiatrist to ask whether a trial course of an antidepressant medication would be worthwhile.

While the foregoing may seem to have ventured far beyond the question of sexual harassment prevention, there is no way to separate what keeps us healthy at work from what keeps us healthy as people. Who we are inwardly underlies how we behave outwardly.

### 5. Hone the Feedback Loop to Recognize What Is Unwelcome

Once a man becomes reasonably aware of his own patterns of fantasy and makes a conscious effort not to base his outer behavior on them, managing his sexual boundaries becomes a much easier task. Indeed, he may develop rewarding and useful interpersonal skills that extend beyond the particular task of avoiding sexual harassment.

The central skill of managing boundaries from the interpersonal point of view is *negotiation*. While many other working conditions are nonnegotiable, and while in some circumstances an individual in authority has the right to impose that authority on others to expedite work, the central principle of boundary management is that everything that has to do with personal space, boundaries, and sexuality is *completely* negotiable. In these situations the imposition of authority is never appropriate.

Because feedback loop skills are the means men have to discover what boundary behavior is unwelcome, honing these skills is essential. Once they stop basing their outward behavior on fantasies, they are free to use their creative masculine intelligence to monitor clues to possible unwelcomeness.

In Chapter 5, when Dave "dropped by" Judy's home insisting that they needed to work on their report that evening, he was imposing authority over both the work that had to be done and Judy's personal boundaries. There is a professional way to handle situations like this, but Dave did not behave professionally. In order to manage the boundaries appropriately, he would have had to do several things differently. First, he would have had to recognize that the whole "dropping by" scenario was being fed by his sexual fantasy. Then he would have had to ask himself if the work really necessitated getting Judy involved that evening.

If the work did have to be done, he would have had to negotiate with Judy the boundary issue of working after hours. He could have called her and said, "Look, Judy, we've got a problem with this report, and I really think we have to take care of it tonight. We need to find an hour. What would work for you? Can you come back to the office, or do you want me to drop over to your house?" This would have given Judy the chance to say, "Dave, it's really difficult, but you're saying, I gather, that we absolutely need to work on it tonight. Is that the case? If I could get a baby-sitter for a couple of hours, I could come in, but I don't think I can find one on such short notice. So why don't you come over here at eight o'clock? I'll clear a space at the kitchen table."

This is a true negotiation. Dave is being adamant that the work needs to be done tonight, but he is letting Judy determine how it is to be done. Even though working at her home is still a boundary crossing into her intimate space, it now has a completely different character. First, he has essentially asked for Judy's permission to drop by, as opposed to springing it on her and offering no options. Next, he has allowed her to set some boundaries, even within her intimate space. She is able to name the time of arrival and prepare a work space with its own good boundaries, the kitchen table.

The very act of negotiation implies respect for another person's boundaries. All Dave needs to do now is to continue allowing her to control the boundaries within her personal space. He must recognize that simply being at her house has created a sensitive boundary issue and that he has to make an extra effort to come at the agreed-upon time, to sit at the kitchen table, to engage in no extraneous chit-chat, and to leave when the work is finished. He does not have the option to suggest they move to the living room couch or have a drink afterward. Actually, once he sets aside his fantasy scenario, a truly professional handling of the boundary issues should follow easily.

Of course, not all men have sexual fantasies brewing in their interactions with women at work. When they do not, there should be fewer obstacles to negotiating personal boundary issues with the utmost respect. When a man does harbor a fantasy, however, he must recognize its presence, then set it aside.

### WHEN YOU ARE NAMED IN A COMPLAINT

Artie, a forty-five-year-old family man, worked as a pole-climbing repairman for a cable television company. He came to see me after Ellie, a woman on his crew, filed a sexual harassment complaint against him. He was depressed and seething with anger, feeling she had betrayed him. He had had only one moment of weakness with Ellie, he said, when he had embraced and kissed her in the cab of his truck after a late-night repair during a severe storm. After bravely climbing the pole under dangerous conditions and restoring service to a whole section of his city, Artie had felt like a bit of a hero. Although he was married, he had long been attracted to Ellie, and when he held her that night in the storm, it had felt well deserved, and he had been sure the feeling was mutual.

But Ellie told a different story. She felt that Artie had previously made a number of comments about how much her body appealed to him. She pointed out in her complaint that he outranked her on the crew and outweighed her by a hundred pounds. According to Ellie, she was so surprised and fatigued the night Artie kissed her that there was little she could do about it. But it certainly hadn't been welcome.

The union was providing Artie with legal counsel, and the company's human resources department had referred him for counseling. As I discussed the situation with him, it became clear that although he was quite ready to admit that what he had done was wrong, he felt betrayed because Ellie hadn't come to him directly to clear it up. But underlying his depression and anger was Artie's presumption that because Ellie had brought a formal complaint, he would be forced to tell his wife of the incident. It seemed to me that he was more afraid of this than of the harassment investigation itself.

The company harassment officer indicated that Ellie generally liked and appreciated Artie, did not want him to be severely penalized, and was interested in a mediated apology, on the condition that he let his wife know what happened. Although Ellie acknowledged she had no legal right to ask for this, she told the harassment officer that she thought she would feel safer around Artie in the future if his wife were aware of the incident.

This was, of course, the one thing that Artie did not want to do, and he grew still angrier at Ellie for putting him under this pressure. I suggested to him that honesty with his wife might be justified on its own, as a way of addressing problems in the marriage. I told him I felt it had become a power struggle for him, that he was refusing to do something just because he felt forced to. Moreover, there was every indication that by acceding to this one, admittedly difficult act of informing his wife, he could resolve the harassment complaint with minimal damage to his career.

Artie thought it over, summoned up his courage, and told his wife. She wasn't pleased, but neither was she surprised. She had known something was wrong and was glad to have it acknowledged. From then on, Artie's anger at Ellie diminished. With a more constructive attitude, he took part in the mediated apology with Ellie. She was willing to let the matter drop. While the harassment incident is on Artie's permanent record, there was no other punishment. He is now back driving the repair truck, on occasion with Ellie. And he is committed to working out the difficulties in his marriage.

Although the complaint against Artie was a fulfillment of the nightmare that many men now fear, his case shows that these complaints usually do not arise without cause. Rather, they occur amid the complexity of workplace and family dynamics, where the man's psychological self is an important part of the whole. The intricacies that underlie harassment complaints are likely to offer us important lessons about how to respond to and resolve such incidents without undue escalation.

Sexual harassment complaints have reportedly tripled since the Anita Hill–Clarence Thomas hearings, and the Tailhook and Baker & MacKenzie cases prove that some juries will judge harassment severely. Yet the odds of any one man becoming the object of a harassment complaint are still astronomically low. Some studies have shown that only 5 percent of cases ever reach the formal complaint stage; and nearly all the statistical surveys of sexual harassment incidents show that despite the publicity that sexual harassment has received in the past few years, approximately 90 percent of perceived episodes of harassment are never reported to those in authority.

Nonetheless, men's fear of being charged with harassment reflects their awareness of the new sexual boundaries they are experiencing and the scrutiny to which they are now subjected. It is also true that when men are found to have harassed, their employers, motivated either by fear of their own liability or by genuine interest in promoting a harassment-free workplace, are more likely to impose severe punishment on them, sometimes including job termination.

### You Have Rights: Know Them, Assert Them, and Seek Counsel

How, then, should a man respond if a female co-worker complains about his behavior? First of all, he should remember that he has rights, and that while harassment lawsuits do not have to prove guilt "beyond a reasonable doubt," the high standard mandated in criminal trials, the basic principle of justice that says "innocent until proven guilty" operates in these cases too.

If a complaint is brought against you, you should immediately avail yourself of all the rights to due process that your workplace offers, and you should seek personal legal counsel as well. Unions exist to defend workers' rights, and although in many cases both parties to a complaint are members of a union, your union must still provide you with support and information about how to proceed. Unions can often provide some legal resources as well.

If only a small informal inquiry is being made rather than a formal complaint, it may strike you as arduous or unnecessary to consult a lawyer. But it can save trouble down the line, prevent escalation, and even hasten a fair conclusion to the proceedings, especially if the lawyer has expertise in pursuing opportunities for resolution. Whether operating out in front or behind the scenes in the early stages, an attorney can advise you of your rights and monitor the fairness of the procedures that are being followed. As I see it, asking for a delay even of an informal inquiry in order to collect yourself, regain your psychological balance, and seek legal advice is a sign of professionalism, as well as a demonstration that you have good boundaries of your own. Properly trained sexual harassment officers at workplaces and on campuses should be sensitive to your wanting to retain legal counsel and even help you obtain it, rather than pressure you into making premature disclosures.

Regardless of whether a harassment charge is or is not valid, no one is served by unclear or arbitrary procedures for investigating it and making a determination about its worthiness. In fact, there is almost always an extended, systematic set of procedures that must be followed. Be sure that the person advising you is knowledgeable enough about these procedures to let you know if the complaint is being handled properly. The sexual harassment field requires specialized knowledge and perceptiveness. For these reasons, human resources or sexual harassment professionals in organizations and schools, and attorneys who specialize in the field, are your best resources.

Appendix A lists some organizations through which you can attempt to find a qualified attorney. Updated information should also be available at the World Wide Web Sexual Harassment Resource site associated with this book.

Another reason it is advisable to seek legal advice is that, rare though it may be, the worst-case scenario in sexual harassment cases is more than just loss of your job and impaired possibilities for future employment—you might be sued for punitive damages for which you would be personally liable, above and beyond any liability on the part of your employer or organization. Admittedly, the percentage of harassment cases that end up in such lawsuits is minuscule. Most never even reach the filing level because they are resolved through the organization's internal procedures; and most cases that are filed are settled before they reach trial. Even when the EEOC pursues a sexual harassment case, extended attempts at conciliation must be made before a lawsuit can be filed. But because the "nightmare" scenario *can* occur, it is important for you to do what you can to protect yourself legally. Unless your counsel advises you to persist and dig in for a courtroom battle, many avenues are usually available for mediated resolution of sexual harassment complaints.

## Do Not Contact Your Accuser: Use Third-Party Negotiation

When a human resources or other workplace officer approaches you informally about a possible harassment episode, you should see it as an early opportunity to enter a nondefensive, mediating process. While you should seek legal counsel before you describe any of your own behavior to such an officer, except in cases of egregious boundary crossings most harassment issues that begin as gentle, informal inquiries can be resolved if you demonstrate your willingness to deal respectfully *through the mediator* with the person offended, offer an apology for any offense caused, and show a desire to learn why others see your boundary behavior as problematical.

Under no circumstances should you try to deal directly with the person who has complained about you. This will invite suspicion that you might be attempting to silence, intimidate, or retaliate against her. Although Artie felt that Ellie should have come to him directly, he had the good sense not to try to contact her. In the end, she never learned how angry he had been with her.

## Maintain Your Dignity and Professionalism

It hurts to be accused of any impropriety. In addition to issues of career and reputation, being accused of harassment carries a special burden because it is a sexual boundary issue, and implicitly at stake are your personal values and private sexual life, as well as those of the person who has complained about you. The threat of his wife's finding out what he had done was certainly a major roadblock for Artie when he first learned of the complaint against him.

Nevertheless, you should see the possibility that someone will name you in a complaint, however unfairly, as a risk inherent to the work and academic worlds rather than as an unfathomable catastrophe. The more you approach a complaint with dignity and professionalism, despite your inner turmoil, the more opportunity you will have to bring about a sensible resolution.

By accepting complaints and investigations as elements of your working life, you are recognizing that the organization you are part of has a right to create standards and grievance procedures about sexual harassment. You are not, at least at this stage, in the position of fighting your own organization. Your cooperation should reflect well on your general intentions and leave you much more room to work out the complaint through negotiation and conciliation. Heaping anger, invective, or abuse either on your accuser or on the organization will only escalate the problem and block off avenues of negotiated resolution.

Of course, your cooperative attitude assumes that the organization is following fair and equitable procedures. You have both a right and an obligation to yourself to make sure that this is the case and to challenge procedures that are not fair and equitable—again, in a "reasonable," professional manner. It is equally important that your accuser also follow the proper procedures and not try to damage you through innuendo or punish you outside the process. If she is, counsel should by all means advise you how to deal with it. If she proceeds improperly, it may actually undermine any legitimacy in her initial complaint.

Unless you are advised by an attorney to behave otherwise, I would suggest that you maintain a professional, cooperative, problem-solving stance at all times in a sexual harassment investigation. Your openness to a conciliation process, rather than a counteraccusatory defensiveness, should reflect well on you.

### True Versus False Accusations

The archetypal nightmare is the false complaint. But even here, common sense indicates a nondefensive, respectful, cooperative attitude (subject, of course, to the advice of legal counsel). You have nothing to hide and you are dismayed that this is happening, yet you wish to offer whatever assistance you can to get to the truth of the matter. If you don't fan the flames unnecessarily, the hope is that a false or baseless complaint will fail on its own merit. It would be wonderful if matters always worked out according to the truth; unfortunately, this doesn't always happen, and true miscarriages of justice do occur. But the chances of such injustice occurring should markedly diminish if one proceeds in a professional manner.

Often a complaint has *some* truth to it, although there can be enormous differences in interpreting how serious the boundary trespass actually is. At other times a man knows that he has indeed stepped over the line. In both instances, once again, the sooner a professional, negotiating, and cooperative stance is taken, the better the outcome should be.

There are many levels at which a harassment complaint can be resolved, as some of the examples already given indicate. Even though Tom engaged in a major, if not egregious, boundary crossing when he put his hand on Linda's thigh, they were able to work it out completely on their own. The elusive healing moment can happen when two people create it together. Unfortunately, the realities of the workplace are such that this kind of resolution is rare; remember that Tom and Linda were equals and had a creative partnership at work. Even people who are equals, such as Ed, the neck-rubber, and Winnie, may need the intervention of a mediator to resolve the complaint. The majority of boundary crossings involve people of at least some unequal authority, and in these cases mediation is even more important.

### Don't Create Monsters: Get Psychological Support

As uncomfortable as it is to have to deal with a sexual harassment complaint, remember that in all likelihood your accuser is sincerely pursuing her rights as she understands them. Although at a deep psychological level the "monster" scenarios may be operating overtime for both people in a harassment complaint, it is important to remain outwardly civil, professional, and respectful of your adversary. If she perceives you as trying to make her into a monster, she may try to do the same to you, and that can escalate the situation. Artie was on the verge of doing this with Ellie; fortunately, he was able to put a stop to it by telling his wife about his indiscretion.

Harassment investigations are stressful, and it is important to have the psychological support of people close to you at such times. Psychotherapy may also help during the crisis. It is very important not to let your feelings affect your outwardly professional demeanor. In this psychologically traumatic event, you need a setting in which you can give voice to your sense of vulnerability, outrage, and, if need be, even hatred about what is happening to you. Therapy can also enable you to discover new inner resources, learn how to enter negotiations in a more flexible way, come up with specific strategies for resolving the problem, and deal with whatever losses may result from the complaint. In the end, the resolution of the complaint against Artie involved addressing some deeper issues in his life that he had neglected over the years.

## WHEN MEN ARE HARASSED

Unusual though it may be, men are also subject to being sexually harassed. The popular imagination got a strong dose of this scenario in Michael Crichton's novel *Disclosure* and the film that was made from it. Although the audience was privy to the truth about the sexual advances of the character played by Demi Moore, what emerged was a film less about female-male sexual harassment than about the false-accusation charges that the Michael Douglas character had to endure.

Men can be harassed either by another man or by a woman in a true reversal of the usual pattern. The identical standards apply in both situations: to be harassing, the behavior has to be sexual in nature and unwelcome; it must either be part of a sex-for-jobs (quid pro quo) arrangement or lead to a hostile working environment. Observation as well as numerous studies note that when women begin acting sexually with men in the workplace, men are much less likely to experience it as unwelcome than when a man comes on to a woman. Men, because of their physical capabilities, traditional positions of authority, and cultural conditioning, are far less likely to feel physically or psychologically coerced if a woman approaches them sexually.

Nevertheless, harassment by women can and does happen. Ned was referred to me for consultation after Wendy, his boss in a small realty office, kept insisting that they conduct business meetings after hours at a local cocktail lounge. On one occasion Wendy drank more than usual and reached under the table for Ned's genitals. He did not find this welcome and brushed her hand away. But over the next few weeks, she scarcely spoke to him at work. When Ned finally decided to broach the subject of what happened in the cocktail lounge, Wendy said, "I don't want to discuss that.

And by the way, I think we're going to have to lay you off—business has been awfully slow lately." Ned consulted an attorney, who suggested that he file an EEOC complaint for quid pro quo harassment.

Men can also be subjected to anti-male gender harassment, such as when a woman supervisor makes anti-male comments or otherwise shows a pattern of discrimination on the basis of his gender. The EEOC guidelines apply here as well. The conduct is considered harassment if it is unwelcome and "has the purpose or effect of unreasonably interfering with an individual's work performance or creating an intimidating, hostile, or offensive working environment."

## THIRD-PARTY SEXUAL HARASSMENT

Both men and women can be victims of so-called third-party sexual harassment. If someone gets a job or promotion ahead of you because he or she has an intimate relationship with the person making that decision, it is discriminatory behavior toward you on the basis of sex and is considered a form of sexual harassment.

## EMPATHY AND ETHICAL VALUES IN SEXUAL BOUNDARY BEHAVIOR

Other than fear of legal consequences, there is another reason that men might question their boundary-crossing behavior with women. It grows out of the direction in which I believe the ideal of the Reasonable Man is developing: toward internalized ethical values. Ethics provide a framework for making decisions based on values that are not mandated by law, but are instead accepted internally by an individual as a matter of common decency and of participation in the values of the community.

Is it asking too much of men to make an ethical decision not to subject women to sexualized behavior, even when they can be fairly certain they will not be disciplined for it? I don't think so. Once men begin to question their own sex-role upbringing, which has usually included a significant dose of sexually opportunistic behavior that leads away from true intimacy, they are likely to discover their own natural capacities for empathy and compassion.

Empathy is the next feedback loop skill beyond reading a woman's boundary messages accurately to know whether what one is doing is welcome. Empathy enables a man to read or imagine what a situation must feel like to the other person. It allows a man to surmise or perceive that women, even those lacking good control over their sexual boundaries, are not really engaged in sexual fun and games.

Insofar as men have been pushed toward unempathic, stereotypical, and predictable responses to sexual situations with women, they too have been devalued. One reason why the field of sexual harassment is so important, not just legally but as a matter of ethics and values, is that it offers both genders an opportunity to step away from damaging caricatures and discover their individual selves.

Another way for a man to think about the ethical aspects of boundary behavior is to imagine the respect he would want the men around them to accord to his teenage daughter, sister, niece, wife, or other loved one. If this standard of respect is fairly stringent, it could serve as a model for the man's own behavior toward the women he encounters. The touchstones of that standard are ethics and compassion.

As Charley, a recent MBA graduate who went to work for a major corporation, told me:

> I went out with this secretary from work the first week I was there—she was one of those "easy" women that you can spot with your radar if that's what you're looking for. We went to bed a few times, then I didn't ask her out again. She quit the job—I'm sure it's because she didn't want to face me at work. So she got hurt piled on hurt. I'm not sure I could do that again. Maybe if I *knew* I wasn't taking advantage of her—but I know I was. I'm just beginning to imagine what it would feel like if I were vulnerable to being used like that.

Ethics and empathy are intertwined aspects of the same issue: becoming more aware of the deeply unconscious patterns that drive men and women to continue reenacting dysfunctional sexual boundary scenarios with each other. Sexual harassment law is one way that our society has chosen to address what might be seen, more fundamentally, as an ethical problem.

Perhaps recognizing the illegality of sexual harassment is a prelude to agreeing, in our hearts and in our behavior, that it is unethical as well.

As time goes on and, in Judge Beezer's words, "the standards of reasonableness change," I believe that men whose ethical values are offended by other men's sexual behavior will become the most powerful role models of all and crucial factors in the prevention of sexual harassment. The new Reasonable Man is already emerging, bringing with him major changes in the accepted sex-role behavior of men. Mirroring the Reasonable Woman, the Reasonable Man will in the end do more than anything else to protect men from the nightmares of a sexual harassment complaint.

We all want to feel that we control our own sexual boundaries and that no one can violate them either by physical force or by the threat of economic loss or physical intimidation. Because as a rule men control their sexual boundaries without any serious threat that they will be violated by force, they have more room to enjoy the intrigue and fantasy excitement of a woman approaching them sexually. Women do not yet have that luxury. True gender equality will be in place when men and women are equally safe, equally in control, and equally playful should they wish to be. It is a day to look forward to.

As it is now, when a man's position and control over his own destiny are threatened, he will, as he should, fight very hard for his rights. Women want to be able to do the same.

# 7. A GUIDE FOR WOMEN

*Taking Charge of Boundaries and*
*Initiating a Complaint*

Despite all the officially stated sanctions against unwelcome sexual behavior that our society now affords women, a woman's guardianship of her sexual boundaries is still very much in her own hands. While enlightened laws and sexual harassment policies tell you as a woman that you have rights of redress if your boundaries are crossed, they haven't yet created a world where you can expect these boundaries not to be constantly tested and challenged. Thus, preventing sexual harassment means, among other things, taking control of your own boundaries. Even if the power equation often favors the man, every boundary problem is still a two-person interaction, and any assertiveness skills you can bring to bear on a potential harassment situation may make a world of difference, not only in the outcome but in how you feel about yourself.

In order to develop such boundary skills, most women must combat well-entrenched gender-role conditioning that discourages them from exercising control over their personal and physical space and that has often punished and endangered them when they have attempted to exert that control. In this chapter we first discuss the difficult psychological issues involved in asserting boundaries and reporting sexual harassment; then we outline a series of practical steps to deal with boundary incursions and harassment.

To be sure, some women are already in firm control of their boundaries. They move about in the world of men with relative ease, exercising the skills necessary to deal with sexually harassing behavior: verbal reprimands that set limits, powerful nonverbal expressions that let men know when to back off, the ability to move away from a situation where they do not feel comfortable, a talent for spotting masculine sexual boundary game-playing, and a willingness to use official complaint channels when necessary. Whether they were taught good boundaries as children or have gained them through hard work and conscious effort as adults, these women not only have necessary boundary-setting skills but, even more important, feel an internal sense of *permission* to assert themselves in a man's world.

Yet all too many women in our society have been systematically discouraged from asserting healthy control over their boundaries. A great deal of research documents that from the early grade-school years on, many teachers, parents, and other role models reward girls for being deferential and pleasant in situations of interpersonal conflict and discourage them from making physical and verbal demonstrations of their anger. Sadly, it is precisely that anger, channeled into verbally assertive social skills, that could enable girls to grow up with both the means and the permission to protect their boundaries.

As matters have stood, it is boys who are usually given permission to be physically and verbally demonstrative of their anger, and they are often accorded prestige for just these qualities. From early school years onward, girls who express their anger in ways that are accepted as normal for boys tend to be labeled as "unladylike," as misfits, or in even more demeaning terms, as "bitches" or "dykes." As a result, preadolescent girls learn either to submerge their expressions of anger in favor of the peer-group standard, or they continue their "unladylike" ways and suffer from being labeled as deviant.

As Emma told me during a consultation about a sexual harassment incident at the rent-a-car counter where she worked:

> I absolutely hated it when my supervisor first started patting my rear as he walked by me, but at first I was totally incapable of saying anything to him, and I hated myself even more for that. I'd ignore it and at the end of the day just smile at him and leave work quickly. It was just like at home, where my father was the boss. It's not that he ever touched me in the wrong way. It's just that whatever he said or did, that was it and there was no

discussion. My mom learned to placate him, to coax him with her smiles away from being angry.

But one day at work, I don't know what happened, but suddenly I just blew up at my supervisor when he patted me while I was waiting on a customer. I turned around and bellowed, "Stop that!" I just couldn't hold back—it's the first time in my life I ever exploded at anybody. It worked in a way—now he won't even come near me and hardly speaks to me. But now he's started messing around with my schedule, giving me more of the lousy shifts than anyone else. That's why I'm thinking about filing a harassment complaint. But no matter what happens to the job, I feel really good about what I did.

As Emma's story shows, the same deference that girls learn as they grow up can be reinforced in workplace harassment. Men such as her supervisor count on the reluctance of women to engage in open conflict in order to continue their boundary violations. But once Emma did speak out and defy the unwritten rule that she suffer in silence, her supervisor seems to have decided to punish her for her "deviance." At the time I saw her, I felt that her psychological liberation from the need to placate would equip her to fight against the retaliation she was experiencing from him.

## BECOMING CLEAR ABOUT YOUR OWN BOUNDARIES
### AND SEXUAL MESSAGES

The proliferation in our society of men's fantasy images of sexually available women also heavily conditions girls as they grow up to learn sexually stereotypical behavior rather than boundary-setting skills. Not only pornography but even mainstream movies and television are replete with women who purportedly live to fulfill men's sexual fantasies. These fantasy images of what women ought to be place women in double danger. First, unless they are strongly repudiated at home and in the community, girls will tend to adapt to the stereotypical female roles that are all around them; and second, even if they do begin to resist by taking better command of their boundaries, they will still find themselves in a society in which men are used to asserting sexual boundary control. The result will be sexual harassment and other forms of sexual imposition on the part of men who have little internal motivation to implement less aggressive boundary behaviors.

According to law, to sexual harassment policies, and to common decency, a woman is not to blame if a man misreads her signals and inflicts unwelcome sexual behavior on her. Regardless of how a male co-worker reads your sexual availability, he has the responsibility not to attempt a sexual boundary crossing. When you are one-to-one with a man, whether at school or at work or on a date or a social occasion, the law won't be there to help you, but you can help yourself enormously if your feedback loops are alert to two typical kinds of interactions. In the first, the man you are with is actually receiving sexually encouraging messages from you, even when you think you are concealing them. In the second, the man has decided, based on his fantasy life, that you would welcome sexual behavior from him, although you are sending no such signals at all.

Combating unconsciousness about such interactions can be a complicated process and involves developing two kinds of awareness: an awareness of what you *intend* to communicate about your sexuality, its potential availability, and where you draw your boundaries; and an awareness of how men around you are reading those messages. At times there can be a troubling discrepancy between what you wish to communicate and the sexual boundary messages that men are receiving from you—often because men have a stronger tendency than women to interpret nonsexual behavior as sexual. These differences in perception can result in anything from a mild, easily remedied misunderstanding to an egregious act of sexual harassment.

Here is how sending unintended sexual messages occurred for Jodie, who worked as a receptionist for a group practice of six male doctors. A female colleague of mine who saw Jodie in therapy told me this story:

> Jodie came to see me during her lunch hour for help in dealing with one of the doctors at work. He would brush against her when they passed each other in the narrow halls leading to the examining rooms, and he'd hang out at her desk, making idle chatter, near the end of the day. A few weeks after our sessions began, Jodie reported that on the afternoons after she saw me, this doctor would always escalate his behavior, lingering over her

desk and, she was sure, staring at her breasts. She found him creepy, but he had done nothing too overt, so she didn't want to jeopardize her job by making an issue of it.

Ever since this behavior had begun, she had felt depressed, scared to go to work, and frustrated with herself for finding herself in this mess. My sense was that her depression would be eased if she felt less powerless over what was happening with this man.

I had also wondered why Jodie said that the doctor seemed to harass her more on the days after our meetings than on other days of the week. I had noticed that for our therapy sessions, she always wore a business suit with a sheer white blouse under a black blazer jacket. I asked whether she wore this same outfit to work every day. No, she said, she didn't—she only wore the suit and blouse on the Wednesdays that she came to see me; on other days she was likely to wear baggier clothes and sweaters.

This was a delicate matter, but I told Jodie I had noticed that when she took her blazer off, the outline of her nipples was sometimes visible through her blouse. She flushed scarlet, reached for her blazer, and said she had no idea that this was happening. Back in the office on Wednesdays, did she also remove her blazer? She said she did. Since it was likely that the doctor might in fact be looking at her breasts, I asked if she had any idea of how much seeing the outline of a woman's nipples can stimulate a man and his fantasy life. She told me that she usually tried to avoid thinking about such things, but that it sounded reasonable to her, and she was glad I had brought it up.

I didn't see Jodie for a few weeks, and when she returned to my office, I could see that her depression had visibly lifted—in fact, until this session, I realized I had never before seen her smile. She proudly informed me that she was now choosing her clothes more carefully, and that our discussions had also motivated her to take great care with this doctor not to show any friendliness beyond what she felt was strictly professional.

Although she reported the happy result that the doctor had ceased his brushings and staring, it was clear to me that what was even more important to her was the fact that she now felt a newfound power from within that allowed her more control over her boundary interactions.

Admittedly, the doctor had no right to make boundary incursions on Jodie, whatever she wore and whether or not she was aware of its effect on others. The standard of behaving nonsexually toward people unless you have confirmation of welcomeness does not change because of the way a woman dresses. Yet it is very much to a woman's advantage, easing depression born of helplessness, to know as much as she can about any signals she is sending out that might be interpreted sexually, and to be able to adapt her behavior accordingly.

## WOMEN IN CONTROL OF THEIR BOUNDARIES

A woman who is in control of the sexual boundary messages she is putting out can participate in the feedback loop at a conscious level and make adjustments as necessary. Della, a young woman who worked as a rep for a medical supply company, spent most of her working day making sales calls at business offices and meeting with the men who decide whether to buy her company's products. She explained her experience of sexual boundary tension in this way:

> Most days I just don't want to deal with the sexual games that a lot of my customers play. I wear a business suit with baggy trousers. I put my hair up, and I don't wear much makeup. I'm pretty careful about being really to the point when I talk, and not being overly chatty. I mean, with some men, all you have to do is say one little thing about the weather, and there they go with some flirtatious comment. If I say it's cold out there, it's, "I'm glad you came in here where I can warm you up." If I say it's warm, they go, "Let's cut work and go cool off together." They can take any sign of being friendly as an excuse for thinking you're interested in them. So I'm real careful. I'm not saying all guys are like this—I also run into a lot of perfect gentlemen

at work. When I'm talking with them, I never feel like parts of their minds are probing me, checking me out sexually while they're talking business.

But once in a while, maybe my hormones are up, or I just feel adventurous, or there's a guy on my route that day I kind of like. So I'll wear a short skirt, or one with a little slit, and a blouse with a button open. No cleavage or anything slutty, but I know it's different from usual. And so do the guys on those days. They *really* want to chat. They stand closer to me. They want to walk me through more doors, all the way back to my car, and unless I make a quick getaway, they just want to keep me there.

I don't know whether or not I sell more product when I'm being more sexy. I should chart it and see. It takes more energy to deal with all their flirtatiousness on the sexy days. But I really don't mind. After all, dressing that way is my choice, and I'm in control of it, so I feel fine about doing it. I don't care if I lose a sale because a guy's unhappy with my not playing games with him. And I also have the advantage of being able to leave a situation whenever I want to and get in my car. It wasn't as easy when I worked in an office every day. If there was a guy being creepy around you, you just had to put up with it unless he really stepped out of line. I think I've learned, since there's no escaping that lots of men are playing sexual games all the time, at least to play the game more on my own terms.

Della is operating out of a conscious awareness of the day-to-day messages between men and women as they monitor and test sexual interest and sexual boundaries. She understands and accepts that many of the men she deals with have an undercurrent of sexual fantasy that affects their behavior toward her. She doesn't try to change that; instead, she has learned how to work with it. Della seems very plugged into the feedback loop, and she can adjust her own behavior if she feels uncomfortable about the way a man is relating to her. This strategy may not always save her from egregious boundary crossing; even women with the best boundary and assertiveness skills can be subjected to harassment that is beyond their ability to fend off. But as a rule, she has a fair measure of control over her boundaries. She can even flirt and engage in boundary testing of her own without either indulging in or encouraging unwelcome sexual behavior.

Although some women with Della's sense of control have trouble understanding why other women don't simply say no to men when unwelcome boundary events occur, it is critically important that they retain their empathy for those who do not yet have control over their boundaries, so that they can act as mentors and positive role models.

## MEN'S RESPONSES TO WOMEN IN CONTROL OF THEIR BOUNDARIES

Many men respond more respectfully to women who are in control of their sexual boundaries than to those who are not. Paradoxically, this remains true even if a woman at times decides to flaunt rather than hide her sexuality, as Della admitted she sometimes does. The key element in the masculine response is not the degree of overtness or sexiness the woman displays, but the degree of authority over herself and her boundaries that she projects.

There are exceptions, of course. Some men feel that a woman in control of her boundaries is challenging his traditional male control over both his boundaries and those of the women in his world. Men like these may work even harder to try to "break" a woman who seems authoritatively in control. If such a man fails, he may then resort to hostile anti-feminine rhetoric: The woman is a "cold bitch," a "lesbo," for whom he has the right prescription: "Someone ought to just take her and screw her brains out."

Hostility toward a woman in control is also evident in retaliatory behavior against women who have brought sexual harassment complaints. In 1995, when the Chevron Corporation agreed to settle for $2.2 million a harassment lawsuit brought by four women, the more serious charges against the company were of egregious retaliation against these women for their having filed complaints about harassing behavior. After it became known at Chevron that one of the women had brought a complaint, she began receiving e-mail containing violent pornographic descriptions. And in a terrible waste of male ingenuity, one man was able to program the computer network so that, when the women booted up their computers in the morning, the initial "greeting" onscreen was a depiction of a man masturbating.

## MEN'S RESPONSES TO WOMEN WHO ARE NOT IN CONTROL OF THEIR BOUNDARIES

For women who cannot or do not exert control over their boundaries, the hazards are greater. A woman like Jodie, who is unaware of the sexuality she is awakening in the men around her, is at increased risk. It is as if men have a radar for sexual energy that such women unconsciously "leak" into their surroundings. Doug, an airline pilot I interviewed, described it this way:

> I think we guys can always tell when a woman seems in charge of herself. You just can't play as many games with her, and you don't try as much, even if you think she's really attractive. You might not like not getting anywhere with her, but there's a grudging respect. Then comes along a woman who may be just as sexy, or even less so, but she somehow doesn't seem aware of what she's putting out. I must admit that's really enticing, because you can sort of pounce on her loose sexual energy, and play around with it. It's hard to describe—as if it's pure sexuality that she's not paying attention to, so you can get to it before she can, and you have the advantage. It might be that you can look her up and down, and she doesn't even notice you doing it. Sometimes you can touch women like this, like in a bar on the thigh, and there will be this pretense that it's just good fun, and even if it doesn't turn into anything, you can feel the electricity in your hand, and everyone's pretending nothing sexual is really happening. You can really take liberties. And you can play lots more games verbally, too, making all sorts of sexual comments, like saying, "I really like to squeeze grapefruits," and they'll let you get away with it.

The phenomenon that Doug is describing is related to the "dumb blonde" jokes and "bimbo" stereotypes that many men seem invested in. It's not hair color or attractiveness or intelligence that they are monitoring, or fantasizing about, in these women. It's a certain quality of dissociated sexuality. A frequent motif in the jokes is that a man is able to trick a woman into having sex. (An extremely mild example: Q. How do you change a blonde's mind? A. Buy her another beer.) As Doug frankly admits, when a woman is not consciously inhabiting her own sexuality, a man feels freer to play around with it.

This feeling of freedom is an ongoing danger to women who are unconscious of their sexual boundaries. If she can't locate these boundaries, how can a woman "live inside them" and take charge of them? And to make matters worse, as Doug notes, men experience a certain turn-on when they encounter a woman like this—it stimulates their fantasies and allows them to take boundary-crossing liberties.

In the old rules, such women were fair game. If they were going to make their sexuality available, men had a right to take advantage of it. In our post–sexual harassment era, however, the rules have changed; they acknowledge that no one should be subjected to this kind of behavior, even if the stereotypes say a woman seems to be "inviting it."

### SEXUAL BOUNDARY PROBLEMS BEGIN AT HOME

Because many women are still locked into sex-role stereotypes that produce exactly what Doug described as being so enticing, those who don't consciously inhabit their own sexuality not only allow men to take liberties with it but lack the psychological know-how to define this behavior as unwelcome. A demeaning and at times abusive heritage deprives many women of the ability to control their sexual boundaries; then men ridicule them as dumb blondes or bimbos and blame them for bringing sexually aggressive behavior upon themselves.

The pressures on girls to adapt to these sexualized cultural messages are exerted most strongly in close or intimate settings—especially by the men in their personal world. How fathers, uncles, stepfathers, brothers, family friends, teachers and other male caregivers behave toward a girl as she grows up will heavily influence her sense of having—or not having—authority over her own body and her sexual boundaries. If they treat her with respect, allowing and encouraging her to set early and continuing age-appropriate boundaries about privacy and how she does and does not wish to be touched, she is much more likely to develop an ability to resist the wider cultural stereotyping and to grow up with good boundary control. Mothers and other female role models are also of central importance in determining the kinds of boundary control and skills girls grow up with. Clearly, a mother who is herself nonassertive about her boundaries will help perpetuate this in her daughter. A mother who resists such stereotyping, however, can teach her daughter to be clear, assertive, and explicit about how she wishes to be treated by men.

When a girl's home setting delivers sexual stereotyping through jokes and sexualized comments, and touching that neither parent opposes, she will have an uphill struggle in adulthood to regain control of her boundaries. Worst of all, if she is overtly sexually abused as a child, she is likely to grow up with an impaired sense of the difference between healthy and abusive sexual touch. This puts her at risk of complying with boundary-invasive behavior as an adult because she simply does not recognize it as such, or of acceding to it because she is too fearful or numbed to object.

Nan, a woman in her mid-thirties, consulted with me on the advice of her attorney as part of a lawsuit against her former psychotherapist, with whom she had had a sexual relationship. As Nan reported:

> For a whole year, Dr. Green was the kindest, most supportive person I had ever met. He simply listened and took seriously everything I said, and I was just beginning to gain a confidence in myself I had never had before. And I was able to tell him about my dark secret—how my brother had come into my bedroom nearly every night when I was twelve and played around with me. But after that first year, I sensed a change in Dr. Green—he started missing appointments and looked stressed out. I asked him if anything was wrong, and he told me that he was going through a difficult divorce. Stupid as I now know it was, I was flattered when he started confiding in me and told me I was the only person in his life he now felt he could talk to about his depression.
>
> One day, he sat there in our session sobbing, then asked me to hold him. I just couldn't say no to him after all he had done for me, and he was so sad. When I did hold him, he then

turned to me and kissed me, quite sexually. Inside I felt numb, but somehow I didn't have the power to say no to him about this either. For six weeks, my therapy sessions consisted of our having sex in his office.

I finally told a friend of mine, who insisted I go see the lawyer, who immediately referred me to a woman therapist. She and I are working on seeing how obvious it is that Dr. Green just repeated what my brother did—he also used to cry if I ever said I'd tell our parents about what was going on. How can it be that the people who are supposed to help you get away from what was sick in your past just get you deeper into it? Even if I can't figure out what a healthy relationship is, aren't they supposed to be able to?

Any woman who has been deprived of control over her sexual boundaries, whether or not the cause was explicit abuse, not only risks sexual harassment and other boundary invasions as an adult. She is deeply traumatized psychologically because the deprivation goes directly to her core sense of self. When a girl experiences her own body and those of other women around her as commodities available for the sexual gratification of men, she is cheated of the chance to feel at one with herself.

All of us measure who we are through our bodies as well as through our psychological selves, and how we feel about our selves is formed in large part by how those around us reflected our value back to us when we were children. If we were fairly consistently loved, valued, and respected both physically and psychologically, we grow up with reasonable self-esteem and an integrated sense of mind and body. If we were invaded, ridiculed, or abused by others, especially by close family members, we are likely to have significant impairments in our self-image and self-esteem.

If people's bodies are objectified, as girls' often are, they can end up feeling split off or dissociated from their physical selves. So helpless do they feel in controlling their boundaries that they effectively cede that control to others, as if their bodies were truly not their own and were thus available to anyone who wishes to take liberties.

Psychologically speaking, many women in our society who have been denied control over their sexual boundaries are living in partially shut-down states that manifest themselves as depressions, dissociations, and fragile, so-called "borderline" personalities. Numerous researchers have shown that these psychiatric symptoms are often rooted in the numbing psychological effects and destabilizing biochemical effects of childhood trauma.

The good news is that the more we understand about the psychological injuries caused by disrespect of boundaries, the more we are able to intervene and enable people to recover from such injuries. Two approaches facilitate this healing: treating people's psychological suffering with respect and understanding, and enabling them to exert power over their social environment so that they will not be continually revictimized.

For such women, seeing a therapist, especially one who provides a positive feminine role model, can be life-changing. Women who have a lingering depression or other problems in which biochemical imbalance may play a part should also consult a physician to judge whether antidepressants or other medications may be of help.

But sound professional treatment, while it can greatly help such women, should not deflect attention from the root causes of their situations and the importance of working to change destructive, pervasive, long-established patterns. Everyone has an obligation not to perpetuate the deeply injurious practice of inflicting unwelcome sexual behavior on others. Men must become equal partners in this effort by breaking with the stereotypical sex-role adaptations that lead them to take liberties with their sexual boundary behavior toward women.

## PRACTICAL STEPS TOWARD HARASSMENT RESPONSE AND PREVENTION

Asserting boundary control in potential or actual situations of sexual harassment involves the following steps:

1. Giving verbal notice
2. Giving stronger warnings and notice that you will report
3. Issuing written warnings and keeping a record
4. Making an informal harassment inquiry
5. Filing a formal complaint within an organization

6. Going outside the organization: filing with the EEOC
7. Going to court

### I. Giving Verbal Notice

When women experience unwelcome sexual behavior, they can assert their right to be treated in acceptable ways through a whole series of stages, from direct interpersonal means to filing lawsuits. The first and probably the most valuable of interpersonal skills is verbal limit-setting.

When a man looks at you, stands too near you, touches you, or says something to you that you do not like, respond with a quick, direct, and simple "I don't appreciate your speaking to me [looking at me] in that way"; or "I don't like your standing that close to me"; "I don't like your touching me." The fact that you have spoken up, asserted control over your boundaries, and served brief, crisp notice about the unwelcome behavior should be enough to deter most men.

Sometimes a followup comment is needed: ". . . and I don't want you to do it again." Not "I *wish* you wouldn't do it again," but "I don't *want* you to do it again." Wishing is too conditional. A wish is something that's not yet true, but what you want or don't want is right here *now*. Because men's boundary behavior is greatly influenced by their "wishes" (that is, fantasies), you don't want to remind a man of the world of wishes. Instead, you need to orient him to the world of *your reality*—by stating what you want and what you don't want, in succinct, explicit terms. This sets a boundary and serves notice of unwelcomeness, all in a few words. There are also less direct verbal means to deal with unwelcome boundary behavior, such as "Excuse me?" said as an expression of objection. This assertion of boundaries and notice of unwelcomeness can sometimes be perfectly effective. But not always; at other times it is less direct than some men require.

Even at this initial level of limit-setting, a man may argue with you or ask what you are talking about when you say, "I don't appreciate that." Even if you are reluctant to get into a debate with him or suspect he will deny the action you are objecting to, you will need to respond with a simple description of what you perceive him to have done.

For instance, you might say, "I don't appreciate your looking at me that way." If he answers, "What are you talking about? I didn't look at you in any way," your answer might be, "It seemed to me that you were ogling me in a way I don't appreciate. If you were, please don't do it again. If you weren't, then it's my mistake and there should be no further problem." Whether or not he is being sincere, you have served notice about unwelcome boundary behavior for the future. "Ogling" is a deliberately bland way of saying "You were looking at me in an offensive, sexual manner." Euphemisms like this are useful at an early stage of trying to establish boundaries and serve notice. They give the man a chance to back down gracefully, and hopefully he will not find it overly accusatory if, in fact, he did *not* actually look at you in the way you thought he did.

Looks, of course, are subject to interpretation. This is less true of actions. When somebody has said something, stood in a certain way, or touched you, your reply to "What do you mean?" should summarize the behavior in question: "You were standing too close to me a minute ago—I don't like that." "You put your hand on my shoulder—please don't do that anymore." "You made a comment about my appearance—I don't appreciate that." "You seemed to be making some sort of sexual comment—I don't appreciate being spoken to in that way." Again, if the man denies it, you can fall back on "It seemed to me that that's what happened, but fine, if it didn't, then perhaps I was mistaken, but I'm sure it won't happen in the future."

For the purpose of working out an accommodation, there is nothing wrong with using the word *please*, as long as you use it in an assertive rather than a pleading way. It is also extremely important not to laugh, apologize, or say "I don't mean to hurt your feelings, but . . ." when you object to the behavior you find unacceptable.

## 2. Giving Stronger Warnings and Notice that You Will Report

If a man's harassing behavior is continuing and your original assertion of notice hasn't changed his behavior, you may want to follow up with another, firmer verbal notice, to the effect: "Look, I don't want this to become a big deal between us, but if it happens again, I'm going to have to discuss this with human resources," or whoever the sexual harassment officer is. If the man argues about whether he did or didn't do anything, whether it does or doesn't constitute sexual harassment, or whether you have any right to tell him how to behave, one way you can respond is to say, "Look, it's obvious we don't see eye to eye about this. Why don't we go see [the harassment officer or someone higher in the hierarchy than both of you] and try working this out?"

During this stage, it is important to do two things simultaneously: (1) assert your boundaries and serve notice of the behavior you find unwelcome; and (2) give the man a chance to back down, gracefully if possible, but in any way at all, even if he is unhappy about it. If he continues objecting, tell him that you are willing to give him one last chance to resolve the incident as if it were a misunderstanding (even if you are privately quite certain that he has knowingly continued his objectionable behavior). At this point you are still trying to reach an interpersonal accommodation rather than report the matter.

### 3. Issuing Written Warnings and Keeping a Record

Along with giving notice about unwelcome behavior, it is important to put incidents of possible harassment in writing as soon as they occur. Even if early-stage verbal notices seem to successfully resolve the matter, you should set down your own private, detailed record of the behavior you found objectionable, what you said or did in response, and when the incidents and exchanges occurred. Ideally, you should make a copy of this record and give it to someone you trust. If you prefer to keep the matter completely private, send a copy of the record to yourself by certified mail, keeping it sealed to establish the date.

There is no way to predict when or how a potential harassment incident that seemed over and done with might resurface, whether in the form of further unwelcome behavior toward you or others, or possible retaliation against you. Should either of these situations occur, you will have a record of the previous events, including documentation of the fact that you already gave this person verbal notice of unwelcome behavior, which you can utilize if a more formal complaint, investigation, EEOC action, or lawsuit ensues.

In the early stages of a possible harassment episode, writing a private message to your harasser, rather than speaking with him, can also be a useful approach. This message should document the behavior you found unwelcome and when it occurred, and request that he stop before you feel it necessary to report the matter. To ascertain that he received it, you can either deliver the note to him personally and ask him to read it in your presence, or ask a co-worker or other third person to deliver it (in a sealed envelope so it remains private) and make certain he reads it. Again, keep a copy for yourself, and note in your record how this written notice was delivered to him.

If the man wishes to talk to you face-to-face about what you said in your note and you feel it is safe and constructive to do so, such an exchange might clear up alleged or real misunderstandings and help you understand each other better. If his response to your note is to become argumentative, however, you should say, once again, that you are still willing to give him a chance to resolve the incident as if it were a misunderstanding. If he should remain argumentative, you may want to suggest that you try to work out your differences with the help of a third person. If his reaction is angry or retaliatory, however, by all means report the incident.

Delivering a note keeps the incident private yet creates a more unambiguous record of notice than spoken notice. It can strongly motivate a man to be more careful about his boundary behavior. From a psychological viewpoint, it is also a means by which a woman can show to herself and others around her that she has control over her boundaries.

## Psychological Readiness, Safety, and the Option Not to Confront

It is often easier to suggest spoken or written responses to early-stage harassment than to carry them out. You may not feel comfortable with delivering a limit-setting comment or writing a note; you may be uncertain that anything untoward actually occurred; or you may simply prefer to ignore the behavior and distance yourself from the person responsible for it. Not taking action is certainly a valid option, and it may be well worth a try, especially if it involves someone, such as a customer, with whom you will not have to do business again. But be wary of relying too much on nonverbal messages, such as physically distancing yourself. While they implicitly assert your boundaries, they may be too vague. Some men need more explicit messages in order to "get it."

As discussed, many women have been reared without the psychological preparation for confronting men about their behavior, and instead socialized to yield control over their boundaries, to avoid interpersonal conflict, and even to doubt their own perceptions of men's behavior. A woman in early-stage harassment retains the right to serve notice, and it is important that she exercise it. It is usually a serious mistake to do nothing at all. If you do not want to confront a man whose behavior you find offensive, and if you find it uncomfortable to clearly signal your distancing yourself from him, you should by all means go to a supervisor or sexual harassment officer and discuss the matter with him or her. Even if you are not ready to initiate a complaint, this officer should be able to give you supportive advice and guidance on how to speak to the man, or discuss with you whether you would prefer to have the message delivered by a third party. Women who are persistently afraid or unable to confront people directly will find counseling, assertiveness training, or a women's support group directed toward this issue very helpful; but these approaches take time. An incident of possible or actual harassment should be dealt with promptly.

One caveat is in order here, with regard to setting spoken or written limits and all subsequent ways of asserting boundaries. In his Reasonable Woman decision (in *Ellison v. Brady*), Judge Beezer noted as a central issue of women's experience that "women who are victims of mild forms of sexual harassment may understandably worry whether a harasser's conduct is merely a prelude to violent sexual assault." Nonetheless, a woman's fear of confrontation can sometimes be so strong that denial may take over even when she feels she may be in actual danger.

If you do sense danger, do not ignore it. Women should always consider their safety first when deciding whether to assert their boundaries directly and interpersonally. If you do not feel safe, don't assert them directly. Go to a third party instead. You may be relatively isolated and not physically safe, or you may simply fear the man's anger and potential retaliation, especially if he is in authority over you. Whatever the reason, respect your instincts. No one else knows what it feels like to be in your position. No one else knows what echoes from your past may be preventing you from feeling safe in confronting someone, or what intuitions of danger in the present you may be picking up.

Do not let anyone, or any messages out there in the world around you, intimidate or shame you into thinking that you have to be heroic and take matters into your own hands. Trust your feelings. If for any reason you don't want to confront, follow your gut feeling and find someone—at work or outside it—with whom to discuss the situation frankly who can offer you guidance on what to do.

Fear of Retaliation and Women's Reluctance to Report

Nearly all statistical surveys on the subject show that approximately 90 percent of perceived episodes of harassment are not reported to anyone in authority in the organization where they occur. Several different factors account for this very troubling statistic.

A woman may be reluctant to report because she is uncertain whether the behavior she has experienced is actually harassment. Let's say her co-worker has asked her out on a date for the third time, despite her previous refusals, and brought her a flower. Even if she feels uncomfortable and wishes he would stop, is she being sexually harassed? She can't point to anything specifically offensive that he has done, and she has never said, "And by the way, please don't ask me again." Nevertheless, she feels she should not be subjected to requests for dates while at work. It is crucial that her organization encourage discussion of circumstances in which the harassing quality of a man's behavior may not be clear.

Diffidence about confronting can also derive from gender-role models that reward girls for conflict avoidance and discourage them from actively asserting control over their boundaries. It may also derive from the differences in male and female relational styles described in Chapter 3. Because women tend to be more interested in mediation and conciliation than in open conflict, they are likely to be reluctant to complain unless an organization's sexual harassment gatekeeper demonstrates genuine respect for these more feminine styles of conflict resolution. Responses to a woman's complaint of harassment should be skilled and flexible, conforming to her wishes to keep it as low-profile as possible. She should be offered an informed perspective on the incident itself, as well as alternative ways to deal with it.

For the woman who has had repeated and unwelcome requests for a date, the harassment officer might suggest appropriate ways for her to talk to him about the issue. Alternatively, the officer could offer to speak directly with the man in a low-key, nonadversarial way. Workplaces in which word gets around that the sexual harassment gatekeeper is sensitive to women's feelings and style will have higher incidences of reporting.

Fear of retaliation—like fear of actual danger from a harasser—is a realistic concern, one that frequently deters women from reporting sexual harassment incidents. Such fear cuts deep. Women's memories of previous punishment, or their observations of what happened to other women who spoke out, have made many of them afraid that they will be subjected to retaliation if they report even a mild incident of sexual harassment. This fear is decidedly "reasonable." Retaliation, a very scary tactic, sends the ultimate double message: Yes, we have laws against sexual harassment and procedures for dealing with it, but we will hurt you if you try to use them. Retaliation can be personal, in the form of more abusive behavior from the man involved, or it can be applied through the organization itself, in the form of undesirable assignments, denied promotions, or even firings.

If the harasser or the organization does retaliate against a woman who brings a complaint, the stakes of the conflict are raised significantly. Permitting such retaliation to occur is a powerful deterrent to an organization's hearing any future harassment complaints. If this kind of retaliation can be demonstrated in court, however, it is such an egregious use of power that it may subject the workplace and the individual named to significant punishment. Clearly, it is essential that organizations send out very strong messages, and back them up, that no retaliation against those who report sexual harassment will be tolerated. This does not eliminate the possibility of covert retaliation, which is a problem when the two parties are unequal in power and coercion is a factor; but it is likely to diminish the frequency of such situations.

Our society is still working out the standards of what constitutes hostile environment harassment. Given the legitimate differences of opinion about this question even at the level of the Supreme Court, we can hardly expect women who encounter day-to-day boundary problems to be able to make a determination of harassment *before* they talk to someone about it. An organization must make it clear that it invites discussion based on *uncertainty,* and it needs to provide skilled people who are able to offer perspective, to educate, and to problem-solve under such circumstances.

An organization that has developed a reputation for flexible, respectful handling of harassment questions in ways that recognize women's styles of conflict resolution, and that has shown that it will not tolerate retaliation, has addressed the major reasons that women are reluctant to report sexual harassment concerns.

## Find the Right Gatekeeper

How does an organization find a sexual harassment officer or other capable individual to help deal with harassment incidents? Medium-sized to large

organizations, and almost all universities, have now recognized the importance of developing sexual harassment resource people who are sensitive to
and respectful of women's boundary issues and the question of direct
confrontation. Educational institutions that receive federal funds (as almost all of them do) must comply with federal sexual harassment law
under Title IX of the Education Amendments of 1972, which prohibits
sex and other kinds of discrimination in educational programs or activities
that receive such funds. (It differs from Title VII of the Civil Rights Act
of 1964, which applies to discrimination in employment.) For this reason,
sexual harassment officers in many colleges and universities are known as
Title IX officers.

In the workplace and in educational settings, such people, whether they
are human resources officers, sexual harassment ombudspeople, or workplace supervisors, are all-important "gatekeepers" whose personal qualities
and skills play a large role in determining whether people who feel harassed
will report incidents more often than they do at present.

Small businesses present more of a problem. Those with fewer than
fifteen employees are exempt from federal sexual harassment laws. State
laws vary—some echo the federal law; others cover businesses with still
fewer employees (see the state listings in Appendix A); and in some states,
notably the most populous one, California, every business is subject to
sexual harassment law regardless of size. It is important to note that the
exemption of small business from federal sexual harassment laws does not
mean that sexual harassment is legal in small businesses. It is illegal, and
legal remedies for such harassment can still be pursued under state unfair
labor practices, or as common law tort personal injury cases (see pages
135–36). But if you work for an exempt employer, it means that federal
EEOC offices and some state agencies cannot intercede on behalf of the
person filing the complaint, and that smaller businesses may not respond
to sexual harassment as well as larger ones do.

Size presents another disadvantage. In very small businesses there may be
no one in authority to whom a woman can speak about a possible harassment incident except the boss himself. And what if he is himself the
harasser? In such a situation, or in any business too small to have its own
internal sexual harassment complaint procedure, a woman will have to turn
to someone outside the organization.

If there is a women's resource center near you or available by phone, it may be able to provide you with perspective on your situation and with information about your options. Organizations sensitive to women's needs have proliferated in the past few decades. Many of them are listed in telephone book Yellow Pages under "Women's Resources"; they can include women's health clinics, battered women's shelters, rape crisis centers, and women's community centers. (Bookstores that specialize in women's issues are found in many large cities and may also be a useful resource.) Although the Yellow Pages may not give specific listings for legal advice about sexual harassment, calling a women's resource organization may lead you to the appropriate person. In towns and cities with women's legal clinics, legal aid societies, or clinics connected to law schools, guidance about sexual harassment should be more readily available. And even if you are not ready to make a formal complaint, the nearest office of the federal EEOC (listed in Appendix B of this book), or its state equivalent, may be able to provide you with or recommend an attorney with whom you can discuss your situation.

In addition, college and university sexual harassment officers are often willing to advise you about resources in your community, even if they cannot directly intervene for you. Because these gatekeepers tend to be quite empathic and knowledgeable, it is worth trying to speak to such a person at your nearest university campus.

Although it might seem like a drastic or expensive step, it is never too early in the process to seek the advice of an attorney who is knowledgeable in the sexual harassment field. Even a lawyer who remains behind the scenes can provide you with feedback on the efforts you are making and the response you are getting, and will be in a position to give further advice if the problem does not head toward resolution. Most attorneys with the necessary expertise are listed as specialists in labor or employment law. Although it may be a challenge to find the right one, the effort is worth it, especially if it should prove necessary to pursue the issue to the level of a formal complaint. (Appendix A provides leads on finding lawyers and other resources. Updated information should be available through this book's World Wide Web Page.)

## 4. Making an Informal Harassment Inquiry

Whether you choose to confront a man about his behavior toward you verbally or in writing, your next step in dealing with a sexual harassment concern is an informal inquiry. Any discussion with a supervisor, human resources person, or designated sexual harassment gatekeeper in which you question someone's treatment of you constitutes an informal harassment inquiry.

At best, this approach can defuse the escalation of day-to-day hostilities and allow those involved to conciliate an incident in a less defensive way. The informal inquiry can lower the risk of polarizing the parties into hostile camps. It is oriented not toward punishment but toward problem-solving, education, and consciousness-raising. This kind of mediation and conciliation is often attuned to women's concerns and styles of conflict resolution.

Nonetheless, although the inquiry is still informal rather than official at this stage, any issue brought to the attention of someone with an official role constitutes a form of serving notice to the organization that there is a problem. Even if that problem is taken care of with minimal discomfort for those involved, the supervisor or harassment officer has a responsibility to make an independent judgment of its possible ramifications. It remains an event of record in the life of the organization, even if no written report is made and if the final determination is that no improper boundary behavior actually occurred.

Conversely, it sometimes comes out in an informal inquiry that a woman was not the first to report difficulty with this particular man, and that he has been put on notice before. The harassment officer or supervisor may also feel the man's behavior is more serious than the woman reporting the problem feels it is. In that case, the officer should give her the reasons for this judgment. The woman may come to agree with it, or she may be able to persuade the officer that her own assessment is the right one. Whatever the outcome, however, the woman should make her own private written record of events, sign and date it, and send it to herself by certified mail or give a copy to someone she trusts.

A private one-to-one discussion is the chief vehicle for an informal inquiry, although under certain circumstances the two people involved in a harassment question may be brought together in the same room for a mediated three-way conversation. A great deal can be accomplished in a face-to-face discussion that is oriented toward deescalation, education, and problem-solving. The experience of human resources officers is that when asked to, most men will end sexual boundary behavior perceived as unwelcome to someone around them.

### 5. Filing a Formal Complaint Within an Organization

At your own discretion, on the advice of the organization's sexual harassment officer, or in cooperation with your own legal counsel, you may decide to file a formal internal complaint. This step raises the issue to a much higher level, where each person in the dispute has more to win or lose. Even if the harassment incident remains within the organization rather than proceeding to the EEOC or to court, someone who is found to have violated his organization's harassment policies could lose his job and suffer serious personal and professional damage.

Once a sexual harassment complaint is reported, it cannot be kept completely confidential. Thus, although those who investigate complaints usually try to maintain as much privacy as possible, in the course of the investigation they may find it necessary to disclose your name and the nature of your complaint, not only to the person you complained about but to others in the organization. Therefore, word that you have brought a complaint may well get out. Some people will admire you for it; others may not. You may find yourself subjected to subtle or overt retaliation or, in rare cases, even to legal counterclaims by the man whose behavior you have protested. If you have not already consulted a lawyer—and as noted above, seeking legal advice is advisable very early in the process—you should certainly do so now. Since the stakes rise when a formal complaint is lodged, it is essential that you have access to legal counsel. The man you have complained about will almost certainly have his own lawyer at this point.

Nonetheless, filing a formal complaint does not automatically mean that a bitter war will erupt. The opportunities and benefits for both men and women that can derive from discussions leading toward a negotiated settlement are substantial. There is still a chance that a more humanizing, deescalating conciliation of the complaint can take place. The goals of consciousness-raising, education, and increased sensitivity—rather than punishment—can still be pursued.

Once you have filed an official complaint, the organization has an obligation to do a fair and competent investigation of your allegations. If it is not equipped to do so on its own, it may contract with an outside consultant or law firm to conduct the investigation, arrive at a determination of what occurred, make a judgment about its harassing quality, and impose a sanction if wrongdoing is found. You will be informed if the investigation determines that your complaint is without merit or cannot be substantiated. In such cases, if you feel that the complaint has not been treated properly, you retain the right to go to the EEOC or to an outside attorney. If, however, a judgment is made that some form of harassment did take place, you may not be informed of precisely what action was taken against the harasser because of his own rights to confidentiality. What you may receive instead is a summary statement that your complaint had merit and that action was taken. On occasion, if you have made a specific request in regard to the outcome—such as asking that the man be transferred or specifying that he attend counseling—the organization may try to implement the request.

In the end, if the organization has done a proper job of investigating and resolving your complaint, the results should be evident: an end to the harassing behavior, an absence of retaliation, and no other signs of a sexually hostile environment. Most women who have been harassed report that their central concern is less the fate of their harasser than whether the workplace becomes safe and harassment free.

Women who move their complaints beyond the workplace, to the EEOC and eventually to state or federal court, usually do so because the organization they work for did not respond adequately to the original harassment charge. In *Ellison v. Brady*, Kerry Ellison sued her employer, not her harasser, claiming that a hostile environment was created when her harasser, after a brief transfer to a different office, was allowed to work near her again, even though he had previously persisted in writing her sexual and scary messages. Judge Beezer found that, given these circumstances, her position might well be reasonable.

## 6. Going Outside the Organization: Filing with the EEOC

Either because a workplace is not equipped to deal with a sexual harassment complaint, or because the complainant feels it has done an inadequate job, a woman may file a complaint with the EEOC (in Canada, the
Canadian Human Rights Commission) or the equivalent state agency. The
EEOC is the federal body that processes workplace violations under Title
VII of the 1964 Civil Rights Act, which banned employment discrimination on the basis of "race, color, religion, sex, or national origin." Many
states also have strong sexual harassment laws and their own equivalent of
the EEOC. (Appendix A lists both the enforcement agencies in these
states, and those that have no sexual harassment laws or enforcement mech-
anisms.)

In filing an EEOC complaint, you are entering a technical area full of
procedural mysteries known only to experts. Although not required by the
EEOC, it is highly advisable that you file under the advice of an attorney
experienced in this specific area. He or she can advise you on how to file
the complaint, and whether to do it with the state or federal agency.
Timing is very important; the statutes of limitations covering the period
between the time of the harassing behavior and the date the complaint is
filed are often relatively brief. The EEOC requires filing within either 180
or 300 days from the date of the alleged harassment incident, depending
on the state where you live.

Such time limits are another reason why it is important to seek legal
advice early in the process. Other complexities need to be addressed as
well, such as whether to file against your organization, your harasser, or
both. Sometimes your nearest federal EEOC or state agency will be able to
recommend an attorney, and under some circumstances it will provide
some funding toward your hiring your own attorney. As mentioned earlier,
legal clinics associated with women's organizations or law schools may be
able to provide services at lower cost.

EEOC offices do not charge for their services, but most of them are
overwhelmed by the number of complaints they receive and are unable to
investigate fully the merits of each one. The most common scenario, therefore, is that after a certain amount of time has passed since you filed (at
least 180 days), you will receive a so-called "right-to-sue" letter from the
EEOC. This simply means that, as required, you have gone to the EEOC

first, which has made no judgment on the case but has cleared the way for you to proceed to the next step if you so decide: suing in a state or federal court. In a very small percentage of cases, the EEOC will decide that your case has enough merit for the commission itself to intervene, first by trying to conciliate the issue with your employer, and at times itself filing its own lawsuit against your employer and/or your harasser.

### 7. Going to Court

Sexual harassment lawsuits tend to be painful, long-drawn-out pitched battles. Since the opportunities to resolve a harassment issue at the prelawsuit phase are usually many, the fact that the matter is now in court means the two sides have polarized instead of drawing toward a settlement. This polarization can come to pass because each party in the suit genuinely believes itself right, or it may simply be that one side hopes it can exhaust the other's time, money, patience, and spirit.

Lawsuits are usually very expensive. If you prevail in a federal sexual harassment lawsuit (known as a Title VII action), or in some state courts, you can be awarded legal fees and punitive damages as well as compensation for lost wages and personal injuries. However, fee recovery is very uncertain, so most sexual harassment lawyers take cases on a contingency-fee basis. This means that the attorney collects no fee if the case is lost or if there is no monetary settlement, or receives a percentage of the award, usually ranging from 33 to 40 percent, when there is a settlement or a jury verdict that imposes a monetary award. Attorneys who work on a contingency-fee basis usually pay all the expenses up front, put in long uncompensated hours, sometimes for years, and risk not recovering a penny. For this reason they are selective about the cases they accept, taking only those in which they feel there is a good chance of financial recovery. At times, law school clinics and women's rights organizations accept cases that they think may establish an important new legal precedent, but this is extremely rare.

Some lawsuits that involve sexual harassment are processed not through the EEOC and Title VII but as common law torts, alleging personal injuries such as assault and battery, intentional infliction of emotional distress, and wrongful termination. Whereas federal Title VII and state sexual harassment suits have strict limits to the amounts that can be awarded, juries in personal injury lawsuits can award large punitive damages. The multimillion-dollar awards in *Weeks v. Baker & MacKenzie* and in Tailhook's *Coughlin v. The Las Vegas Hilton* came from personal injury claims. These actions are filed in state courts, by attorneys who specialize either in sexual harassment as labor lawyers or in personal injury cases. Here too the fee arrangement is usually on a contingency basis. At times it is possible to file a lawsuit that combines Title VII violations and personal injuries in the same complaint.

The defendant in sexual harassment cases, whether an individual harasser or an organization, is usually represented by counsel who is paid by the hour. Some large corporations have tremendous legal resources at their disposal to defend a harassment case. Even these corporations, however, may still be interested in settling, either because they agree that their client engaged in harassment or in order to avoid a costly defense, a large adverse judgment, or negative publicity.

In the end, very few of the cases filed actually go to trial and reach a jury. Most are either settled, withdrawn by the plaintiff, or dismissed by a judge. The settlement process is essentially an extended albeit bitter negotiation resulting in the award of a sum of money that may feel like a victory to either the plaintiff or the defense, that may leave both sides very unsatisfied, or that may, in rare instances, feel to both sides as if justice were properly served.

Becoming involved in an extended sexual harassment lawsuit can dominate a person's life for a long period of time. Because the outcome is so uncertain, my sense is that a woman who is able to sustain such a lawsuit must have more than the possibility of a money award at stake. My wish for women who bring suit is that they feel intensely, win or lose, that there is value in standing up, strongly and in public, for their uncompromised human dignity in a society that has stated that all people have equal unalienable rights under the law.

# 8. A GUIDE FOR ORGANIZATIONS

## *Humanizing the Workplace*

Tim, an assistant manager at a local superdrugstore, tells me, "I got busted at work for supposedly looking too hard at a pretty lady customer. What—now they're reading my mind? The store manager said they'd drop it, but I'll bet I go to the end of the line for promotions." Tim is acknowledging the power that the workplace has to curb what he considers normal male behavior.

Greta, just starting out as a graduate student in hotel management, complains to me that her thesis adviser "tries to cop a feel every time I'm in his office," but then protests, "Bring a harassment complaint about *that?* Are you crazy? Then things would be ten times worse for me. They think stuff like that prepares you for management in the hotel business. And in a funny way, they're right. You just learn to eat it." Greta, like Tim, is also conceding the power that her organization—in this instance, a school— has over her, although in her case she is willing to compromise her personal control over her sexual boundaries.

There is nothing new, of course, about the power that organizations— whether schools, government agencies, nonprofit groups, small businesses, or large corporations—have over our lives, or the relative helplessness we often feel in this regard. What is different today, of course, is the feeling that sexual harassment law has granted *additional* power to schools and workplaces. How can these organizations, many people ask, lay down standards and make judgments about such subjective matters as whether a man has sexual mischief on his mind when he says, "You sure brighten my day," to his secretary, or whether a woman isn't herself engaging in unwelcome sexual behavior by wearing "sexy" clothes to work?

It is certainly true that sexual harassment policies and laws can be used in impersonal and arbitrary ways. As with other kinds of organizational power, abuse does occur. I have seen people on all sides of the harassment issue treated unjustly, sometimes with devastating consequences: completely innocent men unjustly accused, casting a shadow over their lives; women intimidated by harassing behavior at work, then brutalized when they attempt to put a stop to it. Moreover, sexual harassment is not only a new field, it involves complex psychological issues of intimacy, past trauma, and fantasy; so not surprisingly, it has more uncertainty and fluidity than any of the other dimensions by which organizations regulate our lives.

Still, we should not be so carried away by apprehension about the negative consequences that harassment law can and does trigger that we forget that the field represents not just a series of new problems, but also a whole set of new opportunities—for organizations as well as for individuals. This chapter discusses further ways that organizations can allow dialogue to take place, culminating in what I call Reasonable Woman/ Reasonable Man Workshops. Because organizations hold so much power as enforcers of sexual harassment law, they cannot be left to wield that power without our help—that is, without input from the men and women who make up a given organization.

## POLICIES AND PROCEDURES: THE POWER OF THE WRITTEN WORD

The objective of a collaboration between an organization and its members is to allow sexual harassment procedures to be used not as instruments of fear and control but as helpful ways to focus consciousness about sexual boundaries. Any workplace should be able to create dialogues that help bring out the Reasonable Woman and Reasonable Man in all of us. If these dialogues occur on a regular basis, not only after a disaster, then prevention of a sexually hostile environment should be an attainable goal.

The written word is extremely powerful in this context. When an organization distributes the outline of its sexual harassment policy to everyone concerned, it is taking one of the most important steps in changing people's awareness of how to treat one another. As long as no "double message" is being put out by the organization, the harassment-prevention power of distributing a written policy is enormous.

By double message, I mean an unwillingness to back up a sexual harassment policy with action. An organization cannot effectively say, "We posted this policy because the law tells us we have to—but please don't even *think* about bringing us a complaint." A sexual harassment attorney told me about the owner of a medium-sized business who asked his secretary to stay late one night to put the finishing touches on the company's sexual harassment policy. As she sat at the computer, he rubbed her shoulders and told her, "I get turned on thinking about all the things I'm not supposed to do with you. This stuff's all a big joke anyway."

If this man's attitude toward harassment were to leak out to his employees, it would clearly undermine the official policy and invite trouble. Several human resources officers have reported that company chief executives make up a disproportionate number of men who do *not* change when informed that their behavior is unwelcome.

## BUSINESS WARMS TO THE TASK

For this reason, many human resources officers who deal with sexual harassment were delighted by the large jury verdict against the law firm of Baker & MacKenzie. Even if they dreaded the prospect of a similar situation in their own companies, these officers felt that the verdict gave them some leverage with the men at the top. To them, the clear implication of the Baker & MacKenzie verdict was that having a sexual harassment policy in place without taking it seriously was no longer tenable.

"I hate to say this," a male human resources officer told me, "but I've worked at a number of companies where the boss still thinks he can chase the secretary—and tries to hire one he thinks is chaseable. Until Baker & MacKenzie, I had to try pleading to their better natures to stop them from harassing. Sometimes that worked, but I guarantee you that reminding them of a seven-figure jury verdict has been a lot more effective."

Likewise, many corporate attorneys who defend businesses are secretly pleased with the Baker & MacKenzie verdict. They are extremely relieved that such a devastating loss did not happen on their own watch, but they see this case as a historic turning point. They can now go back to the companies whose interests they represent and tell them in no uncertain terms that they must be serious about enforcing sexual harassment policies.

Because almost all of the millions awarded in this case were punitive damages against fellow law partners of the attorney who put the M&M's in Rena Weeks's breast pocket, the verdict is seen as enforcing accountability about sexual harassment all the way to the upper echelons of corporate power.

The good news is that, for the most part, the workplace really is taking seriously the job of raising everyone's consciousness about sexual boundary behavior. Articles on the subject in business magazines are burgeoning. More and more of them, written by human resources officers, attorneys, and sexual harassment consultants, are variants of the same theme: Be sure that you have a sexual harassment policy in place and clear procedures about how to enforce it, and that you send out the message that you are serious about it. Articles about sexual harassment have also appeared in trade journals that serve specific industries—the restaurant business, the consumer electronics industry, and the waste recycling business, to mention just a few—all with suggested outlines of sexual harassment policies that they recommend every business in that industry adopt. Almost all of these outlines begin with this statement: "Inform your employees that sexual harassment will not be tolerated."

In fact, a literature search for sexual harassment articles in business publications reveals them to be far more numerous than in psychology publications. Just as an example, I found twenty-three articles about sexual harassment indexed for 1994 under PsycInfo, a computerized database listing the contents of fifteen hundred psychology journals. In contrast, there were 139 articles on harassment in 1994 indexed in ABI/Inform, a database that lists the contents of a thousand business periodicals.

This is not to underestimate the importance of psychological research, which contributes much to our understanding of the subject. But it does give some indication of where the daily work on sexual harassment is taking place. With employees covered by policies that their companies believe in, and with top leadership kept in check by their own lawyers, human resources people, and the occasional jury verdict, there is cause to believe that the workplace is getting more reasonable by the day about sexual harassment.

## THE POWER OF THE BULLETIN BOARD
## AND OTHER FORMS OF DISSEMINATION

"I've been working for the same construction company for forty years," a bookkeeper named Antonia told me, "and some days I have to pinch myself that I'm not dreaming when I come into work and see those big block letters on the bulletin board about our company's sexual harassment policy. Just because it's up there, I can tell that the men are more respectful of the few girls who work with me. They're lucky. We haven't had a fuss about harassment yet, but I tell you that when I first came to work here, by today's standards I could have filed four complaints every day of my working life!"

What gives Antonia hope does not, in turn, have to cause men in the workplace anxiety. The fact is that everyone will be better protected, either from actual harassment or from a baseless complaint, if a company has a sexual harassment policy and makes sure everyone remains well aware of it. While federal laws do not yet mandate posting such a policy, some states do require it.

Required or not, I recommend that every educational institution, non-profit organization, and business adopt a policy and post it. Sexual harassment policies are not complicated and are easy to come by. (A sample policy is also provided in Appendix C.) Most follow the 1980 EEOC guidelines fairly closely. They begin with that simple assertion, "Sexual harassment will not be tolerated," and go on briefly to define quid pro quo and hostile environment sexual harassment. The next part of the policy should state how and to whom a harassment concern, inquiry, or complaint should be reported. Finally, the procedure for investigating complaints should be outlined, and the possible outcomes.

A policy is a valuable means of accomplishing the most important work in sexual harassment—prevention and raising consciousness. Other steps beyond bulletin-board postings are also worth taking. If a workplace has an internal or publicly distributed newsletter, I recommend publishing an outline of the sexual harassment policy on a quarterly basis for at least a year or two. These periodic, clear and consistent statements about new boundary expectations can counter behavior that has been taught as "normal" from childhood onward in our society. Since the old teachings are deeply embedded in our psyches, the new standards do need reinforcement

over time in order for change to occur. While some people may find
repeated messages that "sexual harassment will not be tolerated" irritating,
even this irritation is a step in the process of internalizing new values.
Bryce, a man of twenty-eight who works on the assembly line of an automobile plant, told me:

> All the guys I work with thought this sexual harassment stuff
> was a joke at first—especially because there were only one or
> two women at the plant, and believe me, the language they used
> sometimes embarrassed *me!* But now, every year, we still have to
> have our annual sexual harassment meeting. We hate it—we sit
> there for an hour like sullen schoolkids being chastised while
> they drone on about the policy. Sure, by now we realize that this
> harassment thing isn't going away. But do I have to keep sitting
> through it every year? I'm ready to tell them, "Okay, Okay, I
> give up—I *get* it. Now would you please leave me alone?"

Actually, Bryce's attitude is encouraging. All of us get impatient when
people lecture us about things we already know. But he only knows as
much as he does because at some point in the last few years his company
gave out clear, consistent messages about acceptable versus unacceptable
sexual behavior in the workplace.

## TURNING GLOBAL SOCIAL NORMS INTO LOCAL ONES

Bryce's workplace has established what sociologists call a new "local social
norm." This norm is to be distinguished from a "global social norm." The
1964 Civil Rights Act, the 1980 EEOC sexual harassment guidelines, and
Judge Beezer's 1991 Reasonable Woman decision are examples of global
social norms that established a national policy defining and outlawing
sexual harassment. But as long as these norms remain global, they can seem
distant and abstract, as if they didn't apply to us. In fact, unless our
everyday interactions reflect the new norms, they *don't* apply to us.

The so-called "locker room" mentality is a good example. When Judge
Beezer writes, "We adopt the perspective of a reasonable woman primarily
because we believe that a sex-blind reasonable person standard tends to be

male-biased and tends to systematically ignore the experiences of women," that is a global social norm, on target but lofty. When men in the locker room post a chart of their fantasized ratings of the women in their workplace, that is a local social norm. Clearly the two are in conflict.

It is not nearly as daunting as it may seem to change the deep-seated attitudes men and women have grown up with, or for the organization to convert global into local social norms. For one thing, new global norms cannot be imposed on people by force, fear, or authority alone; for these norms to be accepted, they must ultimately resonate to elements in the human psyche that are receptive to new ways of behaving. For another, nobody is requiring that men eradicate the fantasizing that drives that "locker room" mentality. Men's fantasy spaces can be preserved, but they have to be sequestered. Decades ago, the locker room mentality was a global social norm—men could hoot and whistle and "Hey, baby" women with impunity nearly everywhere. That has now been rejected as discriminatory and harmful, although for a while it persisted as a local social norm. During the last decade, however, as sexual harassment law and awareness of the new sexual boundaries have developed, that local norm has lost its acceptable status as well.

## BOUNDARY WARNINGS AS CARING INTERVENTIONS

As we have seen, 95 percent of men will stop behaving in ways that offend if they are informed about their behavior in private and in a respectful, nonthreatening way. What I believe is happening here goes beyond conveying good and useful information and drawing upon a man's professionalism. When men are told in a one-to-one conversation that someone finds their behavior offensive, they often experience it as a *caring intervention*.

Of course, much depends on the way they are told it, and we must count on an increasingly skilled corps of human resources and other sexual harassment officers to do it well. Even if he or she is motivated by a necessary disciplinary duty, when a human resources officer takes someone aside to alert him to the possibility of sexual harassment difficulties, the man may well realize that the officer is acting in his interest by actively intervening, rather than silently allowing the problem to get worse.

As an example, let's return to the episode of Steve Horner's unwelcome behavior toward Sally Dunheim. When we last heard from them, Betty Culverson, Steve's sexual harassment officer, had called him in to ask him for his version of the late-night office encounter in which he had asked Sally for a "real kiss." At the first meeting with Culverson, Steve had been somewhat defensive, trying to portray Sally as somewhat of a seductress, averring that she was "acting like she was attracted" to him. Culverson did not challenge him at this point. She simply told Steve that she was taking the matter seriously, would conduct a thorough investigation, and then speak to him again in a few days. Steve was anxious about others finding out that he was being investigated for harassment, but Culverson assured him that, while no guarantee of confidentiality could be granted, she would do her best to preserve his and Sally's privacy.

Several days later, as promised, she asked Steve to meet with her again and told him:

> Steve, I know you have put a lot into this company, and you seem to have a great future here. But I must tell you I've concluded that what you said to Sally that night qualifies as sexual harassment. Although no one has a right to treat anyone else in the workplace in that way, the fact that you are Sally's supervisor makes it much more serious. Your thinking that she was attracted to you was not only mistaken, it was irrelevant. I mean, is going up to someone at work and asking them for a kiss any way to go about things even if you *were* right about that person being interested in you?
>
> But I want you to know there's good news here, too. Sally was surprised and hurt by what you did, but she says you've treated her fairly and well at other times, and she values the work relationship with you. She doesn't want this to go any further if she can be assured, not only that you won't do anything like that again, but that you understand why what you did was a serious matter. As for me, although I don't agree with what you did, I appreciate your honesty and cooperation with me. I judge you to be somebody who is already learning a lot from this in a positive way. I'd like it if you'd have a few counseling sessions with a therapist who knows something about sexual harassment. After that, if there are no further

problems, I think we can put this aside. How does that sound to you?

Steve was expecting much worse; he was pleased and moved—not only by Sally's not wanting to escalate, but by the respect implicit in Betty Culverson's manner of handling the situation. He went to his counseling sessions. In all probability, he is one of the vast majority of men who will never repeat their harassing behavior. In my judgment, the kind of learning that occurs when a man is treated in this way goes beyond a shrewd recognition of the need to change his behavior in order not to lose his job. Caring interventions have a positive psychological effect.

Interventions like this can help restore the human dimension in the organization, even when the subject matter is laced with tension—as it certainly is when the issue at hand relates to sexual harassment. Indeed, the fact that stress and anxiety are involved, touching people in their intimate worlds, makes the power of these interventions still greater.

An ethical as well as a legal perspective is involved when organizations maintain the new social norms about sexual boundary behavior. Because fundamental human values are at stake in sexual harassment law, even as it upholds the law an organization may acquire some of the more positive and human qualities that we call community.

## FINDING THAT SPECIAL PERSON: THE CENTRAL ROLE OF HUMAN RESOURCES AND SEXUAL HARASSMENT OFFICERS

Given the considerable stakes inherent in sexual harassment, workplaces and schools should take care to have someone on hand who is both emotionally well suited and appropriately trained to process inquiries and complaints. Publishing and pamphleteering a sexual harassment policy is the easy part. But the people at the center of the sexual harassment storm have to be chosen very carefully. They must have a wide array of skills. Not only must they be fully informed about their organization's sexual harassment policy and procedures, they have to be able to interpret and teach this knowledge to anyone who asks about it. They must keep up with the latest federal and state laws and EEOC regulations. In consultation with the organization's attorneys, they must insure that the harassment policy, along with its grievance and investigation procedures, are in compliance with the law.

All of this knowledge, however, pales in comparison with the human skills that people in this position must possess. They must have the tact of a master diplomat, the mediating and negotiating skills of a first-rate administrator, the empathy and insight of a psychotherapist, and at times the wisdom of a high priestess or priest.

Remarkably, many such people exist. In the business world they often come out of human resources departments. In schools and universities they may be found in counseling offices or in administration, or be drawn from the ranks of the teaching faculty, regardless of their original field—physics, psychology, or horticulture. Ultimately, such a person must have excellent teaching skills and must herself or himself be a serviceable living model of the Reasonable Woman or Reasonable Man.

I therefore exhort every school, business, nonprofit or other agency: Look very hard at the people you already have working for you. The chances are that one of them is well suited to be your sexual harassment officer.

For instance, Maurice, the CEO of a baked-goods company that in the past five years had expanded from one successful store to ten, spoke to me about his sexual harassment officer:

> You know, like every man and every company head, I've been scared stiff of sexual harassment in the last few years. Our business is growing, but one big lawsuit could probably be a knockout punch for us. Not to mention that, with sexual harassment, there is a certain sense of sleaze and shame that we really don't want associated with our product. Believe me, I used to lie awake nights worrying about it.
>
> Originally, because our company was small and there was a "family" atmosphere, I just told people that my own door was always open if anyone felt any sexual harassment was going on. But nobody ever came to talk to me, and I realized that people might not want to talk to the boss. There was a woman named Angela, in my very small human resources department, who I used to bat around some of these gender issues with. She seemed real savvy about it.

Two years ago I asked her if she'd like to be my official sexual harassment officer, half time. She jumped at the chance. Since then, she tells me that two or three people a week come to ask her various questions. We've had one serious problem with a driver who is now on notice that he's gone if he doesn't watch himself, and we had to get our lawyers involved in that one.

But everything else she's handled. I don't know if she's doing therapy, or ministry, or what. But it works. She doesn't tell me the details. I know she's not infallible, but with Angela there, and with the reputation she's built up in the company, I've stopped obsessing about harassment. I guess I'm kind of proud our company can have a resource like this around.

If your organization has no one suitable within, bring someone in from outside. Take good care of them, so that they can take care of you. Pay them well, even if their harassment role is only part of their regular duties. Invest time and money occasionally in sending them to seminars given by law firms or outside consultants, and to professional meetings with fellow harassment officers. Many of the people who do this work, even if they are pleased to be doing it, feel isolated and need to talk to others in their position; after all, they carry with them more knowledge of suffering in the workplace than anyone else in the organization. And because of the special nature of their jobs, much of what they do must be kept in relative confidence, which is an additional burden.

Any organization that locates, trains, and supports the right kind of sexual harassment officer is likely to be repaid handsomely. Obviously, dollars may be saved, in many forms—beginning, most importantly, with the health and well-being of all who work, teach, or study there. In addition, an organization's potential legal liability in case of a lawsuit should be greatly reduced if it can show that it had sensible harassment procedures, encouraged employees to come forth if they had complaints, had a well-trained harassment officer available, prevented retaliation, and carried out its policy with fairness and in good faith.

Networks for locating people with these skills can be found in Appendix A. Because of the rapid development of this field of professional specialization, every effort will be made to maintain updated information on this book's World Wide Web Sexual Harassment Resources Page.

## BRINGING LIGHT AND LIFE TO A SEXUAL HARASSMENT POLICY

Having the right person in this position brings to life the policy posted on the bulletin board or in the company manual. Everyone in the organization should be aware that its harassment officer is available whenever people have concerns about any kind of behavior that might be harassing, whether they are a possible harasser, the object of harassment, or a third party. Although on occasion the officer may have to refer a worker for psycho-therapy, or consult with outside attorneys in order to investigate a harass-ment complaint, the right person in this role can mediate constructively many problems that arise within the organization.

Issues of confidentiality are a major concern of everyone in a harassment inquiry or complaint, and they must be spelled out clearly. Harassment officers will always make an effort to protect the privacy of the people involved, but the nature of harassment situations within the organizational structure, as well as legal obligations, makes it impossible to guarantee confidentiality. This is because the harassment officer has a primary re-sponsibility to intervene with any behavior that might contribute to a sexually hostile environment, as well as to protect the safety of everyone in the workplace.

If an individual is reluctant to talk when informed that confidentiality cannot be promised, he or she should be referred to a therapist or attorney outside the organization. Harassment officers must remain free to use their judgment about consulting with others inside the organization, or with attorneys, whenever this seems advisable, or to warn people or authorities of imminent danger.

Even allowing for these exceptions to confidentiality, a great deal can be accomplished if the sexual harassment officer is someone whom most workers can trust. At times, however, even the most talented harassment officer will be a man when the worker feels she can speak openly only with a woman, or the officer is a woman when a man is needed. At best, an organization will have a backup person or officer of the opposite sex available. Because a woman is much more likely to report harassment when she can speak to another woman about it, every effort should be made to make a woman available to women workers, even if the organization has to contract out for it. The importance of this should not be underestimated—making women feel safer about reporting harassment is a fundamental element in preventing such harassment.

Unfortunately, many businesses are too small to provide the range of services, including both female and male harassment officers, that larger organizations can offer. These smaller businesses need to hire attorneys to serve this function or contract out for a full range of sexual harassment complaint and investigation services in order to make them available to their employees. Specialized personnel-service providers that are available to small businesses are now adding sexual harassment services to their roster. In addition, an increasing number of firms specialize solely in sexual harassment consulting, training, and complaint processing and investigation. Consult Appendix A or the World Wide Web Page for more information about where to find such services.

## REASONABLE WOMAN/REASONABLE MAN WORKSHOPS

Workplace training can make an important contribution to educating executives, managers, and other employees about sexual harassment. This section outlines a seminar that is designed to allow any workplace to answer the core question in the sexual harassment field: What exactly is the kind of behavior that, to a reasonable person, creates a sexually hostile environment?

Because I believe that the only realistic way to answer this question is to ask it of the "reasonable people" in the workplace, and because reasonable women and men are likely to have different views of the answer, I call this training the Reasonable Woman/Reasonable Man Workshop.

This workshop can be taught either by in-house harassment officers or by contracting out to a specialized sexual harassment training organization. Whoever conducts the workshop must have skill in working with both small and large groups. Ideally, it should be conducted by co-leaders (often called facilitators), a woman and a man. A smaller organization might be able to bring all of its personnel to one of these workshops; for larger organizations, the maximum feasible number for any one such event is probably about one hundred.

Before outlining the workshop, let me provide a brief example of the

kind of feelings that will come up in such workplace events when people
are invited to speak their minds:

> Lila Richards and Ben Chalmers, the sexual harassment trainers
> hired by the NorEast Telephone Company, are lecturing on the
> topic of the company's harassment code to a group of 150
> employees, including installers, information operators, tele-
> phone pole climbers, and customer account representatives. Len
> Smith, who has for twenty-five years been driving a NorEast
> cherry-picker truck repairing storm-disrupted lines, raises his
> hand and asks the trainers, "Have they brought you in here
> because they think we're too stupid to know how to treat each
> other?"
>
> As Ben begins to answer, Helena Hernandez, the dispatcher,
> gets up and says, "Len, it's time for you guys to let us tell *you*
> who's stupid around here for a change!" General disorder threat-
> ens to erupt, as Lila and Ben attempt to process the gender
> conflict that has broken out.

Given that people's fantasy lives are central to understanding sexual harassment, it's time to disclose a fantasy I have developed in my years of
working in the field. I believe that our entire society could make rapid
advancements in solving gender gap, sexual harassment, and boundary
problems of all kinds if each workplace would conduct, for half a day once
a year, a Reasonable Woman/Reasonable Man Workshop. The employees
of NorEast Telephone are absolutely ripe for one. In a sense, this is what
Len and Helena were spontaneously trying to create when they interrupted
the more orderly training that Lila and Ben were conducting.

Here is an outline for facilitators of how to conduct such a workshop:

### I. Introduction: Present the Concept of Hostile Environment and Unwelcome Sexual Behavior (about 45 minutes)

Begin as Lila and Ben did, with a concise presentation of the basic elements of sexual harassment law, concentrating on the definition in the
EEOC guidelines, and including your own organization's harassment policies and procedures.

Focus on the concepts of quid pro quo and the hostile environment, and the central idea of unwelcome sexual behavior.

Concede that what is welcome or unwelcome is not always predictable and obvious, because it is based on a feeling that is going on inside another person.

Point out to the participants that:

1. While there are certain skills that we can develop to be more sensitive to what another person feels, ultimately we can't check out every single individual to assess what he or she finds welcome or unwelcome.
2. Instead, we can develop certain general guidelines about what another person might *reasonably* find to be unwelcome behavior that creates a hostile working environment.
3. Those general, reasonable guidelines will probably differ, according to whether the person is a man or a woman.
4. As long as, in their treatment of others in the workplace, people are complying with the general, *reasonable* guidelines that have been established, it is highly unlikely that they will be found guilty of engaging in sexual harassment because of any one individual's *un*reasonable tendency to take offense at what we have done.

### 2. Explain That We Will Create Our Own Reasonableness Guidelines (about 10 minutes)

Explain that the general guidelines of reasonableness are in flux because of larger changes under way in our society about how people want to be treated in terms of sexual behavior.

Other than the egregious behavior that anybody in any setting would find harassing, no one from outside a particular organization can say exactly what, in that workplace and at this time, the general reasonableness guidelines should be.

Therefore, each workplace has to create its own guidelines of reasonable behavior that it expects of people.

### 3. Explain the Structure of the Workshop (about 20 minutes)

Before going into particulars about the workshop structure, lay out two important guidelines:

Court decisions have affirmed that the point of view of the reasonable person should be the standard for assessing whether unwelcome behavior creates a hostile workplace environment. However, there is also a recognition that a woman might reasonably have a different point of view about unwelcome behavior than a man.

Therefore, if a woman is being subjected to possible harassment, the general guideline to use is the perspective of the Reasonable Woman. If a man is being subjected to harassment, then the proper guideline is the perspective of the Reasonable Man.

Tell the participants that the workshop will take about four hours and that the remainder of it is divided into three stages. In the rest of the first stage, lasting about an hour, the women and the men will each develop two lists, to be used when the two groups come together for a discussion session after the lists have been completed. The first list enumerates the behaviors on the part of the opposite sex that everyone in the group finds offensive and wishes would stop. The purpose of the list is to define the Reasonable Man or Woman standard for the organization for the next year. At this stage the list is tentative, subject to modification as described below; but its objective—establishing guidelines for what constitutes offensive conduct—is firm.

The second list each group develops is more venturesome and can be as daring and imaginative as the participants wish: It contains whatever questions, concerns, or statements they would like the other group to respond to. These items can include any subject about the opposite sex that disturbs or mystifies people—including why men (or women) tend to behave as they do. Each group will select a recorder to write down the list as it evolves; a facilitator will check in from time to time to see whether the participants have any procedural questions.

When the groups have created their lists, the next stage of the workshop begins: The two groups come together for another one-hour session in which each reads its list to the other. An open, freewheeling discussion follows under the guidance of a facilitator whose task it is to keep the participants on track.

In the third stage, lasting around thirty minutes, the groups again divide up according to gender to process what happened in the general discussion and to decide whether they want to make any changes in their list of offensive behaviors. Any item that at least ten percent of the participants agree upon qualifies as an offensive behavior, and facilitators should ensure that nothing clearly unreasonable makes it onto the list.

The groups join together once again, announce their final lists to each other, and end the workshop. In closing, the facilitators strongly urge each group to make every effort to live up to the reasonableness standard that the other group has created, even if some disagreements remain. They explain that the EEOC guidelines apply to everyone, but that these lists provide more detail for workers in this workplace than the national guidelines can. The fact that some disagreements remain reflects the reality that men and women differ on what is reasonable, but it is of value for everyone to be aware of what those differences are, even if they cannot yet be resolved.

Finally, the facilitators remind the participants they will reconvene a year from now to revisit these issues and see whether the gap between the two genders' points of view has closed at all. The entire workshop should run a little over four hours.


Workshops like this are not a total fantasy. I have helped facilitate their equivalent several times. To have them become a standard feature at workplaces is an exciting idea. Properly conducted, they would empower each workplace, and the men and women in it, to create their own local social norms, and to conduct increasingly respectful dialogues that would reduce the tension between the sexes; they would prove to everyone that women and men, when asked to do so, can indeed strive toward embodying the hopeful cultural role models of the Reasonable Woman and Reasonable Man.

# 9. OFFICE ROMANCES

## Can Love in the Workplace Succeed?

Workplace intimacies manifest themselves in the same wonderful, vexing, and occasionally even tragic ways as do all close relationships. They can end happily ever after, with two co-workers developing a lifelong intimacy that creates no problem for the organization. Conversely, an office romance that ends with difficulty or distress can bring personal problems into the workplace, causing disruption for the organization as well as for the two people involved. When the two are of unequal power or status, further questions—about either favoritism or subtle coercion—can easily become sexual harassment problems. Finally, although rarely, an individual may become so distraught at the breakup of a workplace relationship that violence becomes a real possibility.

This chapter examines each of the above scenarios, focusing also on the following questions:

1. When should an organization keep out of people's private behavior, and when does it have a right to intervene?
2. When and how does coercion enter the relationship, especially if the two people involved are of different status?
3. Does an ongoing intimate relationship between two people mean that workplace behavior between them can never be considered sexually unwelcome?
4. What about favoritism and other potentially unwelcome consequences to others resulting from a workplace intimacy?
5. What are the dangers, and how can they be avoided, that come with the ending of such an intimacy?

## HAPPILY EVER AFTER: THE IDEAL OFFICE ROMANCE

Tess and Chuck were both twenty-five when they met at the office coffeemaker one day soon after each began work in the customer service department of a large home appliance firm. Although there was a glint of friendly attraction, they went back to their respective phones on opposite sides of the floor and had no interaction for several weeks. Then one day Tess unexpectedly walked by Chuck's desk and offered him a cup of the usual warmed-over office coffee in a styrofoam cup. Chuck thanked her and suggested that tomorrow they go out to lunch together and get some real coffee at a nearby espresso house.

They enjoyed their lattes immensely, laughing together about some of the more eccentric washing-machine owners they had helped in recent days. Matters progressed quickly from there: dinner a few days later, followed by a weekend bike ride and a movie. They dated, became engaged, and were married a year later. Tess was promoted to customer service supervisor, a job she really enjoyed, while Chuck moved up and over to human resources, which was his real interest. They both still work for the company and are happily planning a family.

Yes, the office romance can indeed work out, and it's obviously heartwarming when it does. But it's important to note all that Tess and Chuck had going for them. The most important factor is that they were equals—in official job status, in seniority, in prestige within the company. That, and the fact that their boundary approaches to each other were gradual, subtle, and welcome, eliminated the possibility of coercion. Because neither was in a supervisory position at the time their romance was developing, their personal bond did not raise questions of alliances or favoritism. And because they seemed to be happy together, neither they nor their coworkers were burdened by the consequences of a breakup.

Still, regardless of the happy ending, the question remains as to whether their workplace had a right to intervene in their relationship in any way. Although a few companies have no-dating policies, their legal enforceability is questionable because they limit the right to privacy. In my view, and in that of several human resources officers with whom I have spoken, no-dating policies don't work very well and actually heighten tensions by adding incentives for workers to keep their relationship secret. People who want to see each other will do so anyway. The emotional health of an organization is improved when boundary issues can be discussed openly. When two people in the workplace date, as long as there is no coercion or difference in status between them and the boundary between professional and personal is crossed in a mutually welcome way, it seems to me that they should be able to conduct their private behavior as they wish. As long as their relationship does not disrupt the workplace or raise issues of harassment, it seems unfair to endanger their jobs because they date.

Ideally, a workplace should make it known that it would like co-workers who have ongoing relationships to inform the human resources officer on a voluntary, private basis. When this is done, the officer can intervene more effectively should private tensions between the couple spill over and affect their work performance or impinge on others.

## WHEN WORKPLACE INTIMACIES END: STRAINING THE BOUNDARIES

Not surprisingly, most dating situations fall short of the happily-ever-after scenario. People meet, get to know each other, and decide to move on. Indeed, two workers who are dating but have not stabilized a relationship are entitled to work things out privately. But this process can call for a very delicate balance:

> Leticia and Vic met at the office holiday party, never having seen each other because they worked in different buildings on the sprawling campus of a managed health care headquarters. Although they were of equal job status, Leticia had worked there for eight years to Vic's two, and she was considered to be well connected in terms of company alliances and politics. They saw a lot of each other over the holidays and on New Year's Eve, but thereafter their interest in each other fizzled, and they ended their brief fling by mutual consent.
>
> No one at work had known they were seeing each other, and there was no workplace spillover when they stopped dating because they never ran into each other in the normal course of

their work. But six weeks later Vic was transferred to an office just down the hall from Leticia's. Despite some initial discomfort, they were quickly able to develop an appropriate level of professional interaction, and nobody was ever the wiser about their previous relationship.

At this stage of Vic and Leticia's situation all seemed well, but it is easy to see where potential spillover problems might have developed. They didn't know when they dated that Vic would be transferred to Leticia's workspace. If matters had gone even a little badly between them, it's possible that Vic would have felt he had to turn down the transfer and the new opportunity it represented. Had there been a residue of negative feeling after they parted, Leticia could have felt some elements of a hostile work environment when Vic entered her daily space. Admittedly, without an unwelcome act, such perceptions would chiefly derive from their personal discomfort; but it is easy to see where matters can become fuzzy in situations like this.

For instance, what if five months later either Vic or Leticia approached the other with a request to resume their previous intimacy? Let's say that the one who is approached found the request to be very unwelcome, even outrageous, and wondered, based on their previous shared understanding that the relationship was over, how he or she could have had the nerve to suggest starting it up again. At this point a new boundary-crossing act has occurred, it has happened in the workplace, and it is unwelcome. Has personal discomfort now evolved into a hostile workplace environment? Is this sexual harassment?

My guideline is this: Once people have ended a relationship, they need to revert to the boundary behavior with each other that is appropriate for *all* people in the workplace. The fact of a past intimacy does not in any way validate taking liberties with the other person's boundaries.

Say Leticia approaches Vic, and he feels his workplace has been intruded upon in a hostile way. However mild or strenuous her overture, the rule is still that Vic should give her notice, either directly or through a third party, that he doesn't wish to be approached again. If she persists, her actions may indeed meet the criteria for sexual harassment.

Throughout our "careers" of intimate partnerships, we tend to look back at previous intimate partners with changed feelings. While it's nice to think that a person with whom you once shared intimacy is in some way still dear to your heart, it doesn't work out that way very often. It is human nature to look back at a prior relationship and feel the other person wronged us in some way, even if that wasn't what we sensed at the time.

It isn't easy to resolve feelings of having been wronged in the past, but it can be done. In nonoffice relationships, we are usually able to put some distance between ourselves and the person which allows us time and space to grieve and to develop a perspective on the old relationship. It is harder to do this, however, with an office intimacy, where we must constantly see or deal with the person at work.

For this reason, you may find it helpful to inform a human resources or harassment officer at the very first sign of workplace tension from a previous relationship. He or she can advise, mediate if advisable, and try to anticipate future problems. A workplace that has the right resource individual in place and makes certain its workers know that it welcomes their using such a person when *any* boundary issues arise, is likely to be well repaid—the chances that personal problems will escalate into sexual harassment issues are significantly reduced.

The workplace is also vulnerable to other dangers from failed relationships. The same relationship difficulties that people have elsewhere may be played out openly at work, such as divorces, remarriages, love triangles, infidelities, or the exposure of people's private marital problems. The ultimate workplace nightmare is the spurned lover who becomes physically aggressive, even murderous.

Obviously, stalking and acts of violence go far beyond workplace sexual harassment; so, for that matter, does the exposure of people's private marital problems. Still, boundaries are at the heart of relationship behaviors of all kinds, whether mild or extreme, so a workplace that takes these issues seriously is doing its part to defuse, and possibly prevent, boundary tensions from exploding into sexual harassment or even violence.

## DATING AND INTIMATE RELATIONSHIPS BETWEEN PEOPLE OF UNEQUAL STATUS

Dr. Maria Delsing, one of the brightest graduates of her medical school class, is developing a reputation as a highly skilled resident in orthopedic surgery at Western Memorial Hospital. She is completing her six-month rotation on the team of Dr. Jim Harrison, who has the most successful private practice in the city. Recognizing her potential, Jim has begun making overtures about Maria's joining his practice when her residency ends. Maria, unsure of whether he will choose her or a male fellow resident, asks Jim to join her for a drink late one Friday evening after a particularly grueling day of surgery together. A bit tipsy, she asks Jim to drive her home and makes sexual overtures to him at her apartment. Jim, fifteen years older and recently divorced, politely declines and excuses himself.

Jim phones Maria at home Sunday night and tries to explain that, while he was tempted to respond to her sexual invitation, he is exhilarated by the possibility of her joining his practice and knows that a sexual relationship would both look bad and complicate their working together in the OR. Maria responds that she is embarrassed and appreciative of his frankness and wonders whether they can both put aside her brief moment of seductiveness and go back to working well together. Jim suggests that they can; and Maria realizes after the phone call that her motivation in acting as she had was based more on her anxiety about her professional future than on a personal feeling for him.

The story of Maria and Jim is a cautionary tale. As accepting as I am about dating between co-workers of equal status, assuming that they know the risks and have a resource to tap if trouble strikes, everything changes when the two people are of unequal status in an organization. My recommendation here is very different: Don't do it. People of unequal status or power should *not* become intimately involved with each other. Almost every sexual harassment policy will say the same thing.

The reasons that underlie this difference are discussed in detail in Chapter 5. The risks of subtle or overt coercion developing whenever people of unequal status in an organization attempt to have a sexual intimacy are unacceptably high. If the relationship ends and the work status of the person of lesser power is in any way diminished, it can be difficult not to conclude that the ending of the relationship played at least some part in this change in status.

Moreover, the person of lesser power is likely to have a fairly credible claim that he or she had felt somewhat coerced into the relationship to begin with. Even if this claim is not made, or if it cannot be sustained because during the relationship the intimacy was clearly welcomed, the judgment of the person in greater authority will be open to question for having allowed sexual intimacy to develop within an asymmetrical power relationship.

Coercion is not the only factor involved in these relationships; they also involve conflict of interest. When somebody who is higher in the organizational hierarchy has an intimate relationship with someone lower, it is nearly impossible for the former to make organizational decisions completely free of personal considerations. It sets up a lose-lose situation. Suppose Jim and Maria become intimately involved. If Jim then asks Maria to join his practice, it impugns his motivation, cheats Maria out of knowing that she has earned the role, and lays a basis for a third-party sexual harassment complaint from any other doctor, man or woman, who has applied for the same job. And if Jim does not ask Maria to join the practice, it raises an entirely different set of problems. Is it because he feels uncomfortable about what will happen to their intimate relationship, or because he wants to avoid the appearance of a conflict of interest? Either way, he has cheated both Maria and the practice out of a job she otherwise deserves, and it creates the possibility of her filing a harassment complaint.

The point about conflict of interest is that once such a situation is set up, *anything* a person does to avoid the appearance of a conflict usually gets him or her into deeper difficulties. Showing great wisdom, Jim preserved his ethical ability to make a decision about Maria's career by choosing not to become intimately involved with her.

Of course, people do not always behave wisely, and at times apparently welcome and fully consenting relationships do develop between people of unequal authority. If they are determined to try to make a go of it despite its conflict with company policies, they are of course free to do so. Indeed, I even think they should be helped along in the process, although the organization will be in damage-control mode until the conflict of interest problem is resolved. In rare instances an organization can successfully assimilate an intimate relationship between two people of unequal status; but it demands great openness and goodwill on the part of the individuals involved, and a willingness to submit the problems their relationship raises to the scrutiny of the organization. Clearly, a relationship conducted in secrecy does not qualify. But if the two people are willing to deal with the situation openly, the human resources or sexual harassment officer could examine the issue with them and make recommendations that will defuse potential conflict—as, for example, by shifting the lines of authority.

This open resolution does not happen often, however, and in most situations of unequal authority other procedures are necessary. One way to resolve the risk of coercion or conflict of interest is for one or both of the people involved to leave the organization. But this too can have its costs. If the person in lesser authority quits, others in the workplace are likely to be left with the feeling that the one who remains, who is in a position of some power in the organization, has boundary problems that might spill over to them someday. For this reason it may be preferable that the person in authority be the one who leaves. Although his boundary crossing will not be perceived as sexual harassment as long as it is welcomed by his partner, his decision will be evidence that he has accepted responsibility for putting himself—and the organization—into a conflict-of-interest situation. Of course, if both individuals leave, then they can make a new start elsewhere.

In university departments, religious congregations, and other nonprofit service-oriented agencies, issues of intimate relationships between people of unequal status are often processed as ethical matters by an ethics or professional standards committee, rather than as sexual harassment problems. Still, regardless of the specific authority that handles these issues, in matters of sexuality and the human heart what can clearly be defined according to sexual harassment law extends beyond legal concerns. The question is how we can all learn how to conduct healthy and ethical intimate relationships that sustain, rather than undermine, the personal and the workplace communities of which we are part.

# 10. BOUNDARIES EVERYWHERE

Sitting on the floor of a dorm room with nine college women, Dr. Sheilah Holmstrom, a psychiatrist in her early forties, attempts to maintain a professional demeanor despite her onrushing anger. This is one of three undergraduate women's support groups that she personally conducts as the university's chief sexual harassment officer. Holmstrom is surprised by the strength of her feelings, having assumed that she had developed some degree of immunity after hearing one story after another of forcible sex and date rape, as well as descriptions of sexual approaches that professors, therapists, and clergymen have made to students. But tonight, listening to sophomore Donna Bishop divulge some of the sexual abuse she experienced as a child, she is barely able to suppress her tears. She vows to hold herself together for the next twenty minutes, when she must leave for an emergency meeting with Roland Robertson, the student body president.

Roland has been asked to resign by Barbara Green, chair of the Undergraduate Women's Association, because of rumors that he had been showing pornographic videos in his dorm room. He and Dr. Holmstrom have worked tirelessly on programs to close the gender gap on this campus, and she can't imagine that he would do anything to undermine that effort. As she excuses herself from the meeting, she wonders if bringing about a less hostile atmosphere in the gender wars is an impossible task.

Anyone who recognizes the array of psychological, political, and ethical issues that converge around sexual harassment might well wonder why a person would choose to expose herself or himself to so much turmoil. The answer, for Dr. Holmstrom and growing legions of sexual harassment officers and ombudspeople, lies in the hope that is generated whenever human suffering and conflict are met, heard, and dealt with as "reasonably" as possible.

These people who have chosen to put themselves at the front lines of the harassment and boundary issues are in a sense representing the rest of us. We are all inescapably involved in an unprecedented reconfiguring of the most important rules of daily social behavior—how we treat one another at our sexual boundaries. We are all creating history as we reach for new ways to negotiate those boundaries in the workplace, in our families, and in our private relationships.

## TEACHING HEALTHY BOUNDARIES: CREATING A SAFER WORLD FOR OUR CHILDREN

Sexual harassment is only one of many interlocking elements of this broad reconfiguration of boundaries. We are obviously zealously involved with boundaries when we try to make our children as safe as they can possibly be from sexual abuse, either within their family circle or from strangers on the street. When these children become adolescents, we become passionate in our wish that they develop sexual boundaries that are as healthy as possible in order to avoid the risks, among other factors, of teenage promiscuity, unwanted pregnancy, exploitation by teachers and coaches, date rape, and AIDS. We want them to learn how to have rewarding intimate relationships. And we want them as adults to be free from sexual harassment, degradation, violence, and rape, and from coercion and exploitation by people in positions of special trust.

When we grapple with these matters, we are not only working to create a safer and more ethical world for ourselves and our children, we are serving as a beacon for the generations to come. To the extent that we reach for the Reasonable Woman and Reasonable Man inside us, we have the power to make the world immeasurably safer and saner than the one we inherited.

I am convinced that this vision of a more decent world is what drives people like Sheilah Holmstrom to involve themselves professionally in the

morass of sexual harassment problems: human resources officers, case in-
vestigators, psychotherapists, women's and men's support networks, professors and graduate students conducting research on the problem, and
feminist political leaders and theorists—who, often to their surprise, increasingly find allies in male judges, business executives, and attorneys
working behind the scenes to persuade their corporate clients to create a
harassment-free workplace.

Those who chose to have a professional involvement in sexual harassment got there first. We who learn from them are next. When we draw
upon their expertise as teachers and role models of Reasonable Women
and Men, we are enabled in turn to be guides to our children.

### EACH SEXUAL BOUNDARY ISSUE TOUCHES ON ALL OTHERS

All sexual boundary issues are interconnected. To be sure, not all sexual
boundary problems are equal—there is obviously a world of difference
between, say, sexual harassment and incest. Sexual harassment, even if egregious and proved, is not a felony, while incest and other forms of child
sexual abuse are repugnant criminal acts. Yet there are important linkages
between the two. Both are sexual boundary issues. Both do harm and
disregard the dignity of the individual by invading someone's sexual boundaries.

*What is crucial to understand is that any work that is done to prevent one kind of
sexual boundary offense helps prevent other kinds.* Thus, a family that both practices
and preaches respect for boundaries gives strong permission for its children
to respect and control their own boundaries. Anyone who is taught from
early childhood on to fiercely defend his or her own boundaries will be far
more likely to recognize boundary abuses in adulthood and have the competence to ward them off.

### BREAKING THE CULTURAL-FAMILIAL HERITAGE
### OF UNHEALTHY BOUNDARIES

Conversely, families that have invasive boundary styles will send children
into the world who will accommodate themselves to further invasion be-

cause they barely recognize the concept of boundaries. When such children reach adulthood and do become aware of their sexual boundaries, they are likely to feel that someone else has control over them. Even if they are pushed to the point where they want to defend these boundaries, they will not possess the skills to do so.

The so-called "bimbo" and "dumb blonde" stereotypes discussed in Chapter 7 are examples of how we perpetuate a culture of sexual degradation. They go beyond the failure to teach healthy boundary skills. What we have actually done is teach people explicitly how to give up control over their boundaries so that they will be more available to those who wish to act out their sexual fantasies. Furthermore, adults who have poor boundary skills pass their vulnerabilities down to their children, perpetuating the cycle.

How do we break this cycle? This is where the field of sexual harassment occupies a position of central importance. Even though harassment itself is less offensive than crimes like incest, child sexual abuse, and rape, it has the widest influence and applicability of any sexual boundary issue now before us. Moreover, it is an equal-opportunity issue, relevant to *all* men and women—even to children—regardless of their personal histories, their previous boundary habits, and whatever ingrained attitudes they may have about how men and women behave.

## LEARNING NEW BOUNDARIES THROUGH ROLE MODELS AT WORK

By deciding that sexual harassment in the workplace and schools is illegal, our society has laid the basis for examining boundary behaviors in other settings as well. Although harmful and invasive behaviors in the workplace usually reflect attitudes and beliefs nurtured in families, schools, and communities, it is in the organizational setting that these behaviors are most likely to be challenged today and where awareness of such entrenched attitudes can begin to emerge. Consider the experience of Harriet, a woman who has been brought up to allow people to take liberties with her boundaries, and Blake, a man who has been raised to believe that he can casually put his hands on a woman whenever he feels like it. Both are nineteen years old. As they begin their work careers at a local franchise of a fast-food chain, neither has ever really thought about these patterns.

The company's sexual harassment policy was not mentioned when they were interviewed for their jobs, but they see it posted on the employee bulletin board the first day they arrive for work. Still, Blake conducts himself as he always has, flirting, touching, occasionally commenting on a woman's body. Harriet, at times an object of Blake's "normal" boundary behavior, tolerates it as she always has. When any of the men touch her, say something about her looks, or make sexual remarks, she remains silent, reacting only with the embarrassed smile that she has developed over the years in an all-purpose attempt to ward off other people's anger.

Then a major boundary incident on the job changes everything. One night when they are cleaning up after the restaurant has closed, Stan, a supervisor who Harriet has noticed has careless hands, can't resist giving Erin, one of the waitresses, a pat on the bottom when she bends to pick up a dropped fork. Erin reacts with sudden sharp anger, telling Stan to keep his hands off. The next day, she files an official complaint with the company's sexual harassment officer. Blake and Harriet, who witnessed the behavior, are contacted by the harassment officer and asked to describe what they saw. A few days later, Stan goes on a two-week leave. He returns, resumes his job, and is thenceforth careful about not touching people at work.

It is the first time that Blake's and Harriet's previous experience of sexual boundary behavior in everyday life has been challenged. Although no one has yet reprimanded Blake, he takes notice of what happened to Stan, and he now stops and thinks whenever he starts to touch a woman he works with. He is also more careful about what he says. He even finds he is taking fewer liberties with the women he dates. For her part, Harriet begins to observe Erin's way of moving, her control over her body, her response to people who get too near her. Without articulating what she is doing, Harriet begins to model herself a bit after Erin, to guard her boundaries, to pull back her arm when someone moves to touch it.

What Harriet remembers most vividly is the moment that Erin stood up and spoke angrily to Stan. It had frightened her; she was sure that Stan would haul off and slug Erin or fire her on the spot. She has seen that happen to friends when they try to challenge the men around them. She remembers the day in high school that her classmate Tammy arrived with a black eye. Her father had hit her, Tammy confided, when she asked him to please knock on her bedroom door before he barged in.

But Stan didn't retaliate, and he is now back at work and acting pretty decently. Moreover, Erin went much further than confronting Stan; she used the system, and used it successfully, to change the way she was treated at work. The posting on the bulletin board assumes significance. When Harriet now looks back at Erin's spontaneous boundary-making anger, she begins to imagine herself doing the same thing. A man she has been dating who used to paw at her asks what's gotten into her when she tells him to stop. She decides she ought to date someone else.

As this story makes clear, sexual harassment policies, simply by being clearly posted and appropriately enforced, can indeed be important factors in breaking the cycle of stereotypical, mutually degrading sexual boundary habits. Like Blake and Harriet, reasonable people who have been brought up with these dysfunctional styles can receive powerful wake-up calls when they become part of a workplace that delivers on the basic promise: "Sexual harassment will not be tolerated."

### Delivering a New Local Social Norm . . .

That Harriet could find in Erin a boundary role model is attributable to more than her witnessing Erin standing up for herself. If instead Erin had been retaliated against for defending her boundaries, it would have reinforced the world that Harriet already knew. What allows her to begin internalizing a completely new approach is her experience that the "community"—in this case, the workplace—has made it safe for Erin to speak out. A global social norm that says sexual harassment is illegal has been transformed into an effective local social norm.

Blake went through a similar process. He was able to interrupt entrenched patterns of his own behavior because he saw his workplace upholding the new standard. It also helped that Stan was able to return to work after participating in the harassment complaint process. When a community allows people to change, rather than "breaking" or exiling them for their unacceptable actions, it offers a clear demonstration that there is life after sexual harassment.

### . . . And Putting Reverse Spillover into Action

These are examples of "reverse spillover" in action. Because sexual harassment issues touch us at the core of our intimate selves, they affect us more
profoundly than do other workplace problems and extend into other areas
of our lives. Both Harriet and Blake experienced the positive side of this
spread. The prevailing local social norm their company established spilled
over into their personal lives. As we look into their future, there is reason
to hope that what they learned will allow them to raise any children they
may have with healthier boundaries than they were taught.


## SCHOOL AS CHILDREN'S "WORKPLACE": DEALING WITH PRECURSORS
## OF SEXUAL HARASSMENT

Harriet and Blake's story leads us to a crucial question: How and at what
point do we educate our children about sexual boundaries and harassment?
How did it happen that until the age of nineteen, neither of them had ever
faced the real consequences of the way they had been reared? Will *their*
children go to schools that intervene, from the early grades on, whenever
youngsters began to demonstrate signs of boundary-crossing behavior?

The family is still the most important and powerful influence in teaching children how to control their physical and sexual boundaries. But
school is the "workplace" for children, and it is in school that they begin to
define their view of the social world outside their families. Even boys and
girls who are secure in their boundaries are encouraged when they observe
the school endorsing what they are learning at home. But because it is
normal for children to adopt the values of the peer group, the school that
does not intervene when boundaries are crossed will set up a conflict in
values even for a well-boundaried child.

This problem is obviously greater for children who are not being taught
strong boundaries at home. If a school routinely tolerates boundary incursions, the children have nowhere else to turn, no other models to draw
upon, and they will adapt themselves to the prevailing behaviors—behaviors that are precursors of sexual harassment and other forms of sexual
abuse.

It is therefore very important that from pre-school onward, schools teach and enforce age-appropriate equivalents of harassment-free workplace standards. Girls and boys who are reared with satisfactory models at home will find this reinforced in their classrooms. Those whose homes do not provide them with such models will learn that the community outside has a different, more respectful way of handling boundaries. These youngsters are less likely to accept as "normal" behavior that in the years to come may make them sexual harassers or victims.

### Teaching Harassment Prevention in Schools

Children who have had healthy boundaries modeled for and taught to them early on have an optimal opportunity to internalize these boundaries. The law requires all schools, public and private, to provide a nonhostile environment for their students as well as a harassment-free workplace for their employees. Indeed, our society feels so strongly about protecting minors, who cannot act for themselves, that it has enacted laws that mandate reporting to authorities any evidence of physical or sexual abuse that comes to the attention of teachers, counselors, and child care and health care workers.

Children too can infringe on one another's boundaries, through verbal and physical bullying, threats of violence, and actual physical assault. These behaviors occur in all grade levels, from the early elementary years through high school, and some are actual instances of sexual harassment. In fact, peer sexual harassment complaints and lawsuits based on how children have treated one another in classrooms, in hallways, at recesses, and on school buses have all been successfully pursued. But the mandate imposed by sexual harassment law should not be viewed as a threat. Every school, and the parents, teachers, and children who make up that school's community, should look upon each complaint as an opportunity to teach about healthy boundaries and thereby address aggressive and invasive behavior.

Many schools already have child abuse prevention programs in place that deal with stranger abduction, physical violence, and "good" versus "bad" touch education—issues that were formerly kept under wraps. Programs like these belong in all schools, ideally enhanced with concrete sexual harassment training in age-appropriate language that will help children recognize unwelcome behavior from other children or from adults.

Even fairly young children have no difficulty grasping the ideas of welcome versus unwelcome touch and speech, and they can "get" the concept of the hostile environment if the word *safe* is substituted for *hostile.* I suggest, in fact, that beginning in the fourth grade, schools develop appropriately modified versions of the Reasonable Woman/ Reasonable Man workshops described in Chapter 8. Children are very responsive to group experiences, and participation in sessions like these can actively encourage them to develop their own sense of boundaries and values.

## SEXUAL BOUNDARIES IN ADOLESCENCE

Peer groups reach their peak influence in adolescence, the very period when temptations toward sexual activity are at their strongest. Most teenagers cannot resist adapting to the values of the peer group. At this stage of development, even those with the healthiest boundary messages from home will be drawn toward some form of sexual experimentation.

If the community, as embodied in the school, is going to influence the peer group's values, it must lay the groundwork years earlier and sustain it thereafter. The messages adolescents receive should make it clear that unwelcome sexual advances, physical or psychological coercion, and sexual bribery are all unacceptable. Although this message will reinforce their efforts to control their sexual boundaries, it will still be a continuing struggle—a struggle that will be intensified dramatically if they experiment with alcohol or consciousness-lowering drugs. Because of the risks of HIV infection, the stakes could not possibly be higher. Add to this the barrage of negative examples from peers and from the mass media, and it is obvious that our children need all the help they can get.

Girls in our society face a significant additional pressure. The pioneering research of Carol Gilligan and her associates makes it clear that early adolescence is a crucial time for girls—a point where they are at high risk of submerging their individual strengths, accomplishments, and identities in favor of the more stereotypical roles that the culture traditionally expects of them. Too many girls are encouraged to silence their voices at this age. As Gilligan's studies demonstrate, teachers in the all-important middle-school years tend to favor boys over girls in a variety of ways, calling on them in class more often, tolerating their interruptions, and reproving girls who interrupt.

Our voice is literally one of the most important means we have of controlling our boundaries and setting limits on how others treat us. We must do everything we can to encourage all children to feel safe about using their voices to maintain their boundaries and their self-esteem. This is particularly important in the sexualized atmosphere of adolescence. But because girls are often specifically conditioned not to use their voices, special efforts must be devoted to them; we cannot assume they will speak up without deliberate and frequent encouragement.

## SEXUAL BOUNDARIES ON CAMPUS

Every imaginable sexual boundary issue is in active play on college and university campuses. Young men and women who are just emerging from adolescence and the protection of their families are exposed to whole new worlds—people, lifestyles, worldviews, and ideas that they never knew existed—when they get to college. They relish the academic and personal freedom the university atmosphere provides, but they still look to the institution to provide a safe environment for their explorations.

As we have noted, colleges and universities are obligated by law to provide a high standard of gender equality and freedom from harassment to everyone there—students and faculty members as well as nonacademic employees. There are many interlocking relationships in the community that makes up a campus, and just as many ways to run afoul of maintaining good boundaries. Complicating the picture is the fact that psychologically (and legally for those not yet eighteen), most of the students are in transition from childhood to adulthood.

Thus, in addressing boundary questions that are already complex, universities must give further consideration to whether they should protect students as children or give them freedom as adults. Should there be coed dorms? Can student government have a role in hearing and processing sexual harassment complaints? What can be done about date rape and other forms of coercive sex? Should sexual liaisons between faculty and students be permitted?

#### Preserving Reasonableness: The Role of the "Boundary Specialist"

Given questions like these, every campus needs one or more people like Dr. Sheilah Holmstrom. They may be called sexual harassment or Title IX officers, student advocates, or ombudspeople, but like their human resources counterparts in the workplace, they can more aptly be termed *boundary specialists.* Moreover, all the boundary issues on campus are also felt by the larger society, which in turn often looks to the university for guidance and leadership. The importance of campus harassment officers in helping us understand what constitutes reasonable behavior cannot be underestimated.

With this quest for reasonableness in mind, let's return to Dr. Holmstrom's meeting with Roland Robertson, the student body president who has been rumored to be watching pornographic videos in his dorm room.

> Dr. Holmstrom meets Roland as agreed in the lobby of the student union. She is very relieved to hear Roland tell her that there has been a terrible misunderstanding. There were, in fact, some X-rated videos being shown in his dorm suite, but he had walked in on them and had asked his roommates to turn them off. When they would not comply with his request, he left.
>
> At their meeting, Dr. Holmstrom and Roland agree that the question of showing pornographic videos in a coed dorm should be submitted to the dorm council so that, if necessary, a policy can be established. They note that different rights and considerations must be balanced—the rights to privacy and free expression on the one hand, and the right of students not to be exposed to sexually offensive materials on the other. Roland makes it clear that, although he is personally in favor of barring such material from the dorm because he feels it demeans both men and women, he thinks that the decision should come from the community, not from his personal feelings.
>
> The next day, Dr. Holmstrom reports on her meeting with Roland to Barbara Green, the chair of the Undergraduate Women's Association. While Barbara is not pleased that an order banning X-rated videos from the dorm cannot be enacted

immediately, she agrees that submitting the question to the community is the only procedure to follow under the present circumstances. Barbara is especially glad to learn that Roland feels the way he does about the matter.

Dr. Holmstrom leaves her meeting with Barbara pleased, and a bit more hopeful, that reasonableness has been preserved for yet another day.

## BETRAYALS OF TRUST: FORBIDDEN-ZONE BOUNDARY VIOLATIONS

Boundary issues are in no way restricted to the campus. For instance, the issue of sex between a student and his or her teacher is a subset of "sex in the forbidden zone," which I have defined as a sexual boundary violation by a person who is in a position of trust—such as a doctor, psychotherapist or other health professional, pastor, teacher, coach, or lawyer—and has a responsibility to act in the best interest of the person to whom he or she is providing services.

The ethical codes for most of these professionals, and in many cases state laws as well, oblige the professional not to introduce or allow sex into any of these relationships. Terrible damage is done when a relationship based on trust is exploited sexually, especially by a health professional, psychotherapist, or member of the clergy.

Teacher-student sexual relations are clearly illegal as well as offensive boundary violations when the student is a minor, yet many campuses have been reluctant to enact policies that specifically ban such relations when both parties are adults. Their reluctance rests on issues of consent and the right of association. This point of view says that adults should have the freedom to engage in mutually consenting sexual relationships with other adults of their choosing.

### "Consenting Adults" Versus Abuse of Power

Consent versus abuse of power is one of the leading-edge issues, much debated, through which our society is redefining sexual boundaries. While I agree with the general principle of freedom of association between mutually consenting adults, when one of them has power over the other's academic, economic, or emotional well-being, an element of subtle or overt coercion can be present that undermines the consent.

The defining principles of sexual harassment are useful in clarifying the problem of consent versus coercion. When a student is being graded by a professor, or if that professor is on the student's dissertation committee, and the two are also engaged in a sexual relationship, an implicit quid pro quo harassment scenario is in place, even when the student perceives the relationship as welcome. Moreover, as in the workplace, even when no clear quid pro quo is involved, the inequality of power, and the conflict of interests and motivations inherent in the professor-student relationship, make it extremely difficult to eliminate coercive factors. Sadly, many students who seemingly welcome sexual relationships with their professors look back on them later with a bitter, if belated, recognition that they were taken advantage of.

In my judgment, professor-student relationships fall into the same category as supervisor-supervisee relationships in the workplace, in that a fundamental coercive element is built into them. As sexual harassment law evolved, it assessed the psychological experiences of people in positions of lesser power and found coercion to be present in these relationships.

Consider the experience of Ada, a recent engineering graduate:

> When I got involved with Professor Thomas, I had never been in one of his classes—I had only seen him give a talk on project design at the informal lunchtime series. I went up to him afterward and asked him a question about a point he made, and he suggested I come to his office hours the next day.
>
> I went—I really enjoyed talking to him. He was able to clarify and get me excited about an idea I had for my senior thesis. It's clear we were attracted to each other, and a week later he asked me to go to dinner with him. I really wanted to go but wasn't sure about it. I asked around if there was a policy against student-faculty dating and was told that there wasn't unless you were in someone's class. So I went, one thing led to another, and by spring of my junior year we were living together and he was mentoring me. It was all pretty dazzling and exciting. If anyone

had told me then that students shouldn't be able to date faculty, I would have thought they were crazy.

But just before the start of my senior year, Bob asked me to move out. I could accept that—the relationship was getting rocky, so why go on with it? I finished my senior thesis without his help—it would have felt awkward to have him involved after our breakup. I got an A on it and graduated with honors. But just before graduation, I got rejected for graduate school here. Bob wasn't on the graduate admissions committee himself, but all the professors on it are friends of his.

Several other students were surprised that I wasn't admitted, and they felt it must have been because Bob would have been uncomfortable having a former lover in the department. So I'm suing the department and the university for sexual harassment. I don't feel like I'm the so-called "victim type," although I'm sure they'll try to claim I'm doing this just because I'm a "spurned lover" and that I would have been rejected anyway. I just want a place to continue my work.

I can't say that my relationship with Bob Thomas was "unwelcome." I'm not going to go back on what I felt at the time. It's a strange sort of hidden quid pro quo situation. It's pretty clear to me that if I had never been involved with him, they would have had no reason to turn me down. So what it boils down to is not the usual story where you don't get the job if you don't sleep with somebody. It's the opposite—I don't get the job because I *did* sleep with somebody. Maybe that's a form of retaliation.

What do I think of student-faculty dating now? In an ideal world, it should still be allowed, because people should be able to separate their personal and professional decisions. But obviously they don't. And think of all the power the professor has over your life! As I found out, students are just too vulnerable to some sort of punitive action as a result of a relationship, unless the relationship works out in a completely smooth way, which it usually doesn't. Since this can pretty much be foreseen, I think the university has an obligation to protect our future careers. I think it should be considered unprofessional behavior on the part of any faculty member to date a student.

I agree with Ada, with one exception: Dating and forming intimate sexual relationships between students and faculty should be allowed when power imbalances that come from the fact that one of them is a faculty member and the other a student are truly non existent. The usual scenario would involve a student who is not in a class taught by the professor and a professor who has no authority over the academic career of the student, and the two of them are of similar age and psychological maturity. But even this situation could change in the future. Even when no abuse of authority was perceived when the relationship began, if at a later time this appears to have been a possibility, the faculty member could find himself in an inquiry to determine whether the relationship was sexually harassing or otherwise unprofessional.

Exceptional cases of success, however, do not warrant ignoring the fact that most relationships between people of unequal authority turn out to be disasters—precisely because one or both disregard the psychological coercion built into the relationship.

## FROM SEXUAL HARASSMENT TO DATE RAPE

Although it can happen anywhere, the college campus is a focal point for the problem of date or acquaintance rape. Here the coercion issue is unequivocal. Date rape is rape, pure and simple. Qualifying the term with "date" or "acquaintance" does not dilute the reality that rape has occurred; it only serves to underscore the irony that some people are capable of inflicting this crime on those they know. One would hope that acquaintanceship encompasses the restraint that comes from compassion and caring, making a woman safer in the presence of someone she knows than with an anonymous predator on the street. Sadly, the opposite is often true: Far more rapes are committed by acquaintances than by strangers.

Rape is at the extreme end of a continuum whose initial point is everyday sexual harassment. The dynamics are the same: Propelled by a sexual fantasy, a man, acting out of long-ingrained tradition, allows the fantasy to govern his sexual boundary behavior. In rape the envelope is pushed to its ultimate consequence. Fantasy leads to action. Using physical force and generating a terror that induces psychological coercion, the violent act is imposed upon the other person.

## The "She Really Wanted It" Rape Myth

Much of the time a man is fully aware when a woman does not consent to sex, but decides to follow his own agenda and forces it on her anyway. On other occasions, however, a man replaces a woman's refusal with his own version of reality, and at the moment he truly believes his version—that she wants to have sex with him—over hers. To support this belief, he invokes one of the most common and pernicious elements in the male rape fantasy system: that "she really wanted it."

This pervasive "she wanted it" myth can be imposed before or during the act, or retrospectively, when it is over. An even more destructive myth, repeatedly depicted in movies and on television, says that when a woman is ambivalent or says no to a sexual boundary crossing, she really wants the man to push her a little harder verbally and physically, and then a lot harder. Anyone who counts the number of times a day this scenario is played out on television will be shocked. In an even more diabolical version, a woman who has been fending off a man suddenly changes and participates actively in forced sex. The message here is simple: Applying force at a woman's sexual boundaries will be "rewarded."

## REASONABLE WOMAN/REASONABLE MAN: THE HEALING IMAGE

It may seem strange to move from rape, the ultimate boundary violation, to the idealism of the Reasonable Woman/Reasonable Man. But they are linked more closely than the surface appearance suggests. Boundaries lie at the heart of both, raising the question of whether it is realistic to believe that a society in which sexual boundary incursions are common, and violent sexual assault all too frequent, will be able to change the fundamental patterns that lead to these outcomes.

It is my belief that it can, as is evident both in the law and in the role models on which the law is premised. Progress may be slow, but progress it is. The mandates that make sexual harassment illegal are not very old, yet they have already totally recast the rules of sexual boundary behavior. The recognition is growing that the old gender stereotypes are invalid. The importance of using the school and the community to inculcate respect for boundaries is reflected in the growing number of programs that teach our children these principles. Mediation and dialogue are replacing adversary stances when boundary violations occur. A respected profession committed to preventing and resolving such problems is emerging. All this offers promise that the boundary ideal—and partnership—inherent in the concept of the Reasonable Woman and the Reasonable Man *can* be transformed into reality. Every man and woman who works toward this goal comes ever closer to creating healing moments for themselves, for their children, and for the world in which we live.

# APPENDIX A
# RESOURCES AND
# THE WORLDWIDE WEB

When I began researching this book, I welcomed the fact that my computer had no modem, rendering me safe from what I assumed would be an endlessly distracting entrée into cyberspace. Then it happened: I needed a new machine, and since it had a built-in fax/modem, I warily went on-line. What and whom I found has proved to be immensely valuable: Entire documents about sexual harassment, including some of the most important ones, were instantly available to me. So were answers to questions I put out on Listserv and Majordomo discussion groups; people cheerfully responded through e-mail. If you navigate carefully, there can be a true sense of community on the Internet.

The responsiveness of the on-line community also offered a solution to the problem of resource lists, whose entries may become obsolete in a rapidly changing field like sexual harassment. The resources noted in this book are valid as it goes to press. To keep current, readers have available to them the Sexual Harassment Resources World Wide Web site at http://www.bdd.com/rutter. Through this page, and with the input of others (including readers of this book), I hope to keep available a current list of sexual harassment resources and developments. When you browse it, it will link you to other Web sites worldwide in the same and related subject areas. You may also contact me on the Web site with suggestions, reactions, corrections, or objections to anything in the book written or listed here; or write to me directly by e-mail at pr@itsa.ucsf.edu without accessing the Web site.

The resource lists in this appendix are organized as follows:

**I. Important National Telephone Numbers.** 800 numbers are listed for the EEOC and for women's and men's national organizations; a national number is also given for attorney referrals. Numbers are also given for Canada.

**II. National Organizations.** All manner of information and support is available for both women and men from these organizations.

**III. State Listings.** The first listing under each state is the state agency that enforces sexual harassment law. (For the few states with no such agency, I have listed the local EEOC offices.) Entries for private organizations in the state follow.

These lists have been culled and collated from many sources, including organizations, colleagues, and the Internet. Especially useful were the listings in *Sexual Harassment on the Job: What It Is and How to Stop It*, 2d ed., by William Petrocelli and Barbara Kate Repa (Berkeley: Nolo Press, 1994), and the Web site of the Feminist Majority Foundation **(http://www.feminist.org/911/I__supprt.html)**. I have omitted almost all on-line resources here because they can be found in more current versions on the book's Web site. I am grateful to everyone who helped with this resource list, and I look forward to readers' contributions that should keep the Web site a thriving node in cyberspace.

# I. IMPORTANT NATIONAL TELEPHONE NUMBERS

Equal Employment Opportunity Commission (EEOC): (800) 669-4000 (for referral to nearest EEOC office); (800) 669-EEOC (for procedures and regulations)

Feminist Majority Foundation
1600 Wilson Boulevard, Suite 704
Arlington, VA 22209
703 522-2214 (office)
703 522-2501 (sexual harassment hotline)
Information and referrals
World Wide Web Page:
http://www.feminist.org/911/
I__supprt.html

Men Assisting, Leading, and
Educating (MALE)
P.O. Box 460171
Aurora, CO 80046
(800) 949-6253 (national hotline)
Provides male sexual abuse survivor resources, including sexual harassment; publishes newsletter and organizes annual conference

9 to 5: National Association of
Working Women
614 Superior Avenue
Cleveland, OH 44113
(800) 522-0925 (national job problem hotline)
(216) 621-9449 (Ohio)
Provides information, support, and advice

RAINN (Rape, Abuse, Incest
National Network)
800-656-4673 (twenty-four-hour national hotline)
This hotline will automatically read the area code of the number you are calling from and route your call to the nearest sexual assault crisis line.

American Bar Association
750 Lake Shore Drive
Chicago, IL 60611
(312) 988-5000
Has a local attorney referral service
for both plaintiff and defense lawyers

**In Canada:**

The Canadian Human Rights
Commission/Commission Canadienne
des Droits de la Personne
320 Queen Street
Tower A, 22nd Floor
Ottawa, ON
KIA IEI Canada
(613) 995-1151

Men Working to End Sexism and
Violence
P.O. Box 33005
Quinpool Postal Outlet
Halifax, NS
B3L 4T6 Canada
World Wide Web Page:
http://www.cfn.cs.dal.ca/
CommunitySupport/Men4Change/
m4c__back.html

## II. NATIONAL ORGANIZATIONS

American Federation of Teachers
Women's Rights Committee
555 New Jersey Avenue, N.W.
Washington, DC 20001
(202) 879-4400
Publishes an extensive *Sexual Harassment Resource Guide*

Asian-American Legal Defense and
Education Fund
99 Hudson Street
New York, NY 10013
(212) 966-5932
Has legal assistance and women's
rights projects

Association of American Colleges
Project on the Status and Education
of Women
1818 R Street, N.W.
Washington, DC 20009
(202) 387-3760
Provides bibliographies and other
materials

American Arbitration Association
Center for Mediation
1660 Lincoln Street, Suite 2150
Denver, CO 80264-2101
(800) 678-0823
(303) 831-0823
Offers a sexual harassment claim
resolution process

BNA Communications, Inc.
9439 Key West Avenue
Rockville, MD 20850-3396
(800) 233-6067
(301) 948-0540
Offers training materials about sexual
harassment to large and small
businesses

Business and Professional Women's
Foundation
2012 Massachusetts Avenue, N.W.
Washington, DC 20036
(202) 293-1200
Offers the pamphlet "Crime of Power,
Not Passion"

Center for Women Policy Studies
2000 P Street, N.W., Suite 508
Washington, DC 20036
(202) 872-1770
Offers many publications relating to
violence against women, women's
health policy, and economic
opportunity. See especially *"Friends"
Raping Friends: Could It Happen to You?*
and *Sexual Harassment Action Packet.*

Coalition of Labor Union Women
(CLUW)
15 Union Square
New York, NY 10003
(212) 242-0700
Provides information about the use of
union representatives as sexual
harassment mediators

Equal Rights Advocates
1663 Mission Street, Suite 550
San Francisco, CA 94103
(415) 621-0672 (office)
(415) 621-0505 (information line)
Offers telephone advice in Spanish
and English

Federation of Organizations for
Professional Women
2001 S Street, N.W., Suite 500
Washington, DC 20009
(202) 328-1415
Has workshops and legal fund in
response to harassment

The Men's Health Network
P.O. Box 770
Washington, DC 20044-0770
(202) 543-6461

Mexican American Legal Defense and
Education Fund
1430 K Street, N.W.
Washington, DC 20005
(202) 628-4074
Has lawyer referral service and
regional offices

NAACP Legal Defense and
Educational Fund
99 Hudson Street
New York, NY 10013
(212) 219-1900
Litigates in some sexual harassment
cases

National Center for Lesbian Rights
870 Market Street, Suite 570
San Francisco, CA 94102
(415) 392-6257
Offers legal resources and referrals

National Coalition Against Sexual
Assault
P.O. Box 21378
Washington, DC 20009
(202) 483-7165
Provides information, counseling, and
support

National Council for Research on
Women
47–49 East 65th Street
New York, NY 10021
(212) 724-0730
Offers the pamphlet "Sexual
Harassment: Research and Resources"

National Organization for Women
1000 16th Street, N.W., Suite 700
Washington, DC 20036
(202) 331-0066
Offers information, support, and

publications; 750 local chapters in all states

National Women's Law Center
1616 P Street, N.W., Suite 100
Washington, DC 20036
(202) 328-5160
Provides legal and educational
resources; publications

NOW Legal Defense and Education
Fund
99 Hudson Street
New York, NY 10013
(212) 925-6635
Has legal resource kit for sexual
harassment

Pacific Resource Development Group
Premier Publishing
145 Northwest 85th Street, Suite 103
Seattle, WA 98117
(800) 767-3062
(206) 782-8310
Publishes the Webb Report and other
training materials on sexual
harassment; offers consulting services

Wellesley College Center for Research
on Women
Wellesley, MA 02181-8259
(617) 283-2500
Has extensive publications and guides
regarding sexual harassment in schools

Wider Opportunities for Women
815 15th Street, N.W., Suite 916
Washington, DC 20005
(202) 638-3143
Offers books and support for women
in nontraditional jobs; has a national

tradeswomen resource network of
local organizations

Women's Bureau
U.S. Department of Labor
200 Constitution Avenue, N.W.
Washington, DC 20210
(800) 827-5335
Provides information on rights of
working women

Women's Legal Defense Fund
1875 Connecticut Avenue, N.W.,
Suite 710
Washington, DC 20009
(202) 986-2600
Offers publications

## III. STATE LISTINGS

### Alabama

State agency: none
EEOC Birmingham District Office
1900 Third Avenue N, Suite 101
Birmingham, AL 35203

Mobile Rape Crisis Center
501 North Bishop Lane
Mobile, AL 36608
(344) 450-2244 Office
(344) 473-7273 Hotline

### Alaska

State agency: Alaska State
Commission for Human Rights
800 A Street, Suite 204
Anchorage, AK 99501-3669
(907) 274-4692
(800) 478-4692

Alaska Women's Resource Center
111 West 9th Street
Anchorage, AK 99501
(907) 276-0528

Women's Resource Center Aiding
Women from Abuse and Rape
Emergencies (AWARE)
P.O. Box 020809
Juneau, AK 99802
(907) 586-2977 (office)
(907) 586-1090 (hotline)
Offers support groups, legal advocacy,
education on sexual harassment in
schools

## Arizona

State Agency: Arizona Civil Rights
Division
1275 West Washington Street
Phoenix, AZ 85007
(602) 542-5263

Center Against Sexual Abuse (CASA)
5227 North 7th Street, Suite 100
Phoenix, AZ 85014
(602) 241-9443 (office)
(602) 941-9010 (hotline)

## Arkansas

State agency: none

EEOC Little Rock Area Office
320 West Capitol Avenue, Suite 621
Little Rock, AR 72201
(501) 324-5060

Rape Crisis, Inc.
7509 Cantrell, Suite 211
Little Rock, AK 72207
(501) 663-3334

## California

State agency: California Department
of Fair Employment and Housing
2014 T Street, Suite 210
Sacramento, CA 95814
(800) 884-1684
(916) 227-2873

Asian Immigrant Women Advocates
310 8th Street
Oakland, CA 94610
(510) 268-0192
Provides assistance for women at
work; Asian languages spoken

Center for Working Life
600 Grand Avenue, Suite 305
Oakland, CA 94610
(510) 893-7343
Has support groups, counseling

Defensa de Mujeres
406 Main Street, Room 326
Watsonville, CA 95076
(408) 722-4532 (office)
(408) 685-3737 (twenty-four-hour
hotline)
Provides sexual harassment support
and legal referrals; bilingual

Golden Gate University Law School
Women's Employment Rights Clinic
536 Mission Street
San Francisco, CA 94105-2968
(415) 442-6647
Has employment advice and
counseling hotline

Hastings Law School
Legal Aid Society, Employment Law
Center, Workers' Rights Hotline
1663 Mission Street, Suite 400
San Francisco, CA 94103
(415) 864-8848 (office)
(415) 864-8208 (workers' rights
hotline)
Offers free legal advice to unemployed
and low-income persons only; makes
legal referrals to lawyers who will
represent individuals

Parents for Title IX
P.O. Box 835
Petaluma, CA 94953
(707) 765-6298
Focuses on sexual harassment of girls
in schools; offers support groups for
younger women

University of California, Davis
The Sexual Harassment Education
Program
Guilbert House, 112 "A" Street
Davis, CA 95616
(916) 752-9255 (office)
(916) 752-2255 (anonymous hotline)
Offers information, referrals,
education

University of California, San
Francisco
Women's Resource Center
San Francisco, CA 94143
(415) 476-5836
Makes referrals

University of California, Santa Cruz
Title IX/Sexual Harassment Officer
109 Clark Kerr Hall
Santa Cruz, CA 95064
(408) 459-2462
Offers information, referrals,
education

## Colorado

State agency: Colorado Civil Rights
Division
1560 Broadway, Suite 1050
Denver, CO 80202
(303) 894-2997

Discrimination and Sexual Harassment
Support Group (DASH)
Boulder National Organization for
Women
P.O. Box 7972
Boulder, CO 80306
(303) 444-7217
Has support group; offers legal advice
and attorney and therapist referrals

Domestic Violence Institute
50 South Steele Street, Suite 850
Denver, CO 80209
(303) 322-1831
Offers training, consultation, and
expert witness resources

Rape Assistance and Awareness
Program
640 Broadway, Suite 112
Denver, CO 80203
(303) 329-9922 (office)
(303) 322-7273 (hotline)
(303) 329-0031 (Spanish)

## Connecticut

State agency: Connecticut Commission
on Human Rights and Opportunities
90 Washington Street
Hartford, CT 06106
(203) 566-3350


Connecticut Women's Education and
Legal Fund
135 Broad Street
Hartford, CT 06105
(203) 865-0188 (office)
(203) 524-0601 (information)
Offers counseling for sex
discrimination, legal referrals,
education, and training


Rape Crisis Center
Connecticut Sexual Assault Crisis
Services
(203) 282-9881
Has twenty-four-hour hotline, support
groups, counseling; provides legal
referrals to twelve member centers in
Connecticut


## Delaware

State agency: Delaware Department of
Labor
State Office Building
820 North French Street, 6th Floor
Wilmington, DE 19801
(302) 577-2882


Contact/Delaware
P.O. Box 9525
Wilmington, DE 19809
(302) 761-9800 (office)
(302) 761-9100 (hotline)
(800) 262-9800 (hotline)

## District of Columbia

District agency: D.C. Commission on
Human Rights
2000 14th Street, N.W., 3d Floor
Washington, DC 20009
(202) 939-8740


Federally Employed Women
1400 Eye Street, N.W.
Washington, DC 20005
(202) 898-0994
Provides legal referrals; information
guide on sexual harassment


Trial Lawyers for Public Justice
1625 Massachusetts Avenue, N.W.
Suite 100
Washington, DC 20036
(202) 797-8600
Can provide legal representation


## Florida

State agency: Florida Commission on
Human Relations
325 John Knox Road, Building F
Suite 240
Tallahassee, FL 32303-4149
(904) 488-7082
(800) 342-8170


Family Service Center
2960 Roosevelt Boulevard
Clearwater, FL 34620
(813) 530-7233
Offers counseling; pamphlets on
sexual harassment


Gulf Coast Legal Services
641 1st Street South
St. Petersburg, FL 33701
(813) 821-0726
Offers legal advice

Help Line
(813) 893-1141 (office)
(813) 344-5555 (twenty-four-hour
hotline)
Offers counseling and referrals

Human Relations Department
City Hall
400 South Orange Avenue
Orlando, FL 32801
(407) 246-2122
Investigates complaints in the city of
Orlando

Lawyer Referral Service
(407) 422-4537
Gives listings of sexual harassment
attorneys

The South Florida Sexual Abuse and
Assault Victims Program (SAAV)
5900 SouthWest 73rd Street
Suite 301
Miami, FL 33143
(305) 663-6540 (twenty-four-hour
hotline)
Offers counseling and referrals

Georgia

State agency: Georgia Commission on
Equal Opportunity
710 Cain Tower, Peachtree Center
229 Peachtree Street, N.E.
Atlanta, GA 30303
(404) 656-7708

Dekalb Rape Crisis Center
403 Ponce De Leon Avenue
DeKalb, GA 30030
(404) 377-1428 (twenty-four-hour
hotline)
Offers counseling and educational
services

9 to 5: National Association of
Working Women
250 10th Street N.E., Suite 107
Atlanta, GA 30309
(404) 616-4861
(800) 669-0769 (southeast regional
office)
Offers counseling, legal referrals, and
training seminars

Rape Crisis Center
P.O. Box 8492
Savannah, GA 31412
(912) 354-6742 (office)
(912) 233-7273 (twenty-four-hour
hotline)
Offers counseling, training, legal
referrals

Hawai'i

State agency: Hawai'i Civil Rights
Commission
888 Mililani Street, 2nd Floor
Honolulu, HI 96813
(808) 586-8636 (Oahu)
(800) 468-4644, ext. 6-8636
(neighbor islands)

Office of the Sexual Harassment
Counselor
University of Hawai'i at Manoa
2600 Campus Road, Room 210
Honolulu, HI 96822
(808) 956-9499

Sexual Abuse Treatment Center
1415 Kalakaua Avenue, Suite 201
Honolulu, HI 96826
(808) 973-8337 (office)
(808) 524-7273 (crisis line)

## Idaho

State agency: Idaho Human Rights
Commission
450 West State Street, First Floor
Boise, ID 83720
(208) 334-2873

Idaho Women's Network
P.O. Box 1385
Boise, ID 83701
(208) 344-5738

Women's and Children's Crisis Center
720 West Washington
Boise, ID 83702
(208) 343-3688 (office)
(208) 343-7025 (twenty-four-hour
hotline)
Offers counseling and referrals

## Illinois

State agency: Illinois Department of
Human Rights
100 West Randolph Street
Suite 10–100
Chicago, IL 60601
(312) 814-6200

Apna Ghar
4753 North Broadway, Suite 502
Chicago, IL 60640
(312) 334-0173 (office)
(312) 334-4663 (hotline)
Offers counseling, support groups,
and legal referrals, especially for Asian
women

Pro Bono Advocates
CL88
50 West Washington
Chicago, IL 60602
(312) 629-6945
Offers legal referrals

Women Employed
22 West Monroe, Suite 1400
Chicago, IL 60603
(312) 782-3902
Offers telephone counseling and
advice, legal referrals

YWCA—Women's Services
180 North Wabash
Chicago, IL 60601
(312) 372-6600
Offers counseling, support groups,
and legal referrals

## Indiana

State agency: Indiana Civil Rights
Commission
100 North Senate Avenue
Room N103
Indianapolis, IN 46204
(317) 232-2600
(800) 628-2909

Breaking Free
Indianapolis, IN 46204
(317) 923-4260
Offers counseling and legal referrals

Center for Women and Families—
Rape Relief Center
2820 Grant Line Road
New Albany, IN 47150
(812) 945-0986
(502) 581-7273 (southern Indiana)
Offers therapy, legal referrals, and
crisis intervention

## Iowa

State agency: Iowa Civil Rights
Commission
Grimes State Office Building
211 East Maple Street, 2nd Floor
Des Moines, IA 50309
(515) 281-4121

Rape Victim Advocacy Center
17 West Prentice
Iowa City, IA 52240
(319) 335-6001 (office)
(319) 335-6000 (twenty-four-hour
hotline)
Provides counseling, support groups,
and education

University of Iowa
Women's Resource and Action Center
130 North Madison Street
Iowa City, IA 52242
(319) 335-1486
Provides counseling, legal referrals,
and resources to students and the
community

## Kansas

State agency: Kansas Commission on
Civil Rights
Landon State Office Building,
8th Floor
900 S.W. Jackson Street, Suite 851 S
Topeka, KS 66612-1258
(913) 296-3206

Reno County Rape Survivors Group
1 East 9th
Hutchinson, KS 67501
(316) 665-3630 (office)
(316) 663-2522 (twenty-four-hour
hotline)
Offers counseling, legal referrals, and
education

Sedgwick County, Wichita Area
Sexual Assault Center
215 North Saint Francis, Suite 1
Wichita, KS 67202
(316) 263-0185 (office)
(316) 263-3002 (twenty-four-hour
hotline)
Offers counseling, referrals, and
community education

Sexual Assault Survivors Group
P.O. Box 1526
Manhattan, KS 66502
(913) 539-7935 (office)
(800) 727-2785 (hotline)
Offers support groups, legal referrals

## Kentucky

State agency: Kentucky Commission
on Human Rights
The Heyburn Building, Suite 700
332 West Broadway
Louisville, KY 40202
(502) 595-4024
(800) 292-5566

Center for Women and Families—
Rape Relief Center
226 West Breckinridge Street
P.O. Box 2048
Louisville, KY 40201-2048
(502) 581-7273
Offers therapy, crisis intervention,
legal referrals, workshops

Lexington–Fayette Urban County
Human Rights Commission
162 East Main Street, Suite 226
Lexington, KY 40507
(606) 252-0071
Investigates complaints in Fayette
County

Lexington Rape Crisis Center
P.O. Box 1603
Lexington, KY 40592
(606) 253-2511
Offers counseling, legal referrals,
community education

Louisville–Jefferson County Human
Relations Commission
200 South 7th Street
Louisville, KY 40202
(502) 574-3631
Investigates complaints in Jefferson
County

## Louisiana

State agency: none

EEOC New Orleans District Office
701 Loyola Avenue, Suite 600
New Orleans, LA 70113
(504) 589-2329

Louisiana Foundation Against Sexual
Assault
P.O. Box 1450
Independence, LA 70443
(504) 878-3949

## Maine

State agency: Maine Human Rights
Commission
Statehouse Station 51
Augusta, ME 04333
(207) 624-6050

Augusta Area Rape Crisis Center
3 Mulliken Court
Augusta, ME 04330
(207) 626-3425 (office)
(207) 626-0660 (hotline)
Offers support groups, legal referrals,
training/education for sexual
harassment prevention

Maine Coalition Against Sexual
Assault—Rape Crisis Assistance
P.O. Box 924
Waterville, ME 04903
(207) 872-0601 (office)
(800) 525-4441 (twenty-four-hour
hotline)
Offers support, legal and counseling
referrals, training

Rape Response Services
P.O. Box 2516
Bangor, ME 04401
(207) 941-2980 (office)
(207) 989-5678 (hotline, Bangor)
(800) 310-0000 (hotline, statewide)
Offers counseling, support groups,
legal referrals

## Maryland

State agency: Maryland Commission on Human Relations
20 East Franklin Street
Baltimore, MD 21202
(410) 767-8600

Sexual Assault and Domestic Violence Center
6229 North Charles Street
Baltimore, MD 21212
(410) 377-8111 (office)
(410) 828-6390 (hotline)

## Massachusetts

State agency: Massachusetts Commission Against Discrimination
1 Ashburton Place, Room 601
Boston, MA 02108
(617) 727-3990 (Boston)
(413) 739-2145 (Springfield)

Cambridge Women's Center
46 Pleasant Street
Cambridge, MA 02139
(617) 354-8807
Offers support groups, information, legal referrals

9 to 5: National Association of Working Women
145 Tremont Street, Suite 205
Boston, MA 02111
(617) 348-2970
Offers telephone counseling, educational materials, workshops

Women's Crisis Center
24 Pleasant Street
Newburyport, MA 01950
(508) 465-2155
Offers telephone counseling, legal advocacy, support groups

## Michigan

State agency: Michigan Department of Civil Rights
333 South Capitol
Lansing, MI 48913
(517) 373-3590 (Lansing)
(313) 876-5544 (Detroit)
(517) 373-2884 (Women's Commission)

Women Involved in Giving Support (WINGS)
(810) 437-8091
Offers informational telephone line; legal referrals, support groups in Detroit, Lansing, Kalamazoo, Ann Arbor, and Flint

Women Lawyers Association
(517) 487-3332

## Minnesota

State agency: Minnesota Department of Human Rights
Bremer Tower
Seventh Place and Minnesota Street
St. Paul, MN 55101
(612) 296-5663

Carver and Scott County Sexual
Violence Center
510 Chestnut Street North, Suite 204
Chaska, MN 55318
(612) 448-5425 (hotline)
Offers support groups, counseling,
legal referrals

Chrysalis
550 Rice Street
St. Paul, MN 55103
(612) 222-2823 (office)
(612) 871-2603 (resource line)
(612) 871-0118 (Minneapolis office)
Offers individual counseling, legal
referrals

Sexual Violence Center
2100 Pillsbury Avenue South
Minneapolis, MN 55404
(612) 871-5100 (office)
(612) 871-5111 (hotline)
Offers counseling, support groups,
legal referrals

Washington County Sexual Assault
Services
8200 Hadley
Cottage Grove, MN 55016
(612) 458-4116 (office)
(612) 777-1117 (hotline)
Offers counseling, legal referrals

## Mississippi

State agency: none

EEOC Jackson Area Office
Cross Road Building Complex
207 West Amite Street
Jackson, MI 39201

Rape Crisis Line
P.O. Box 2248
Jackson, MS 39225
(601) 366-3880 (office)
(601) 982-7273 (hotline)
Makes legal referrals

Gulf Coast Women's Center
P.O. Box 333
Biloxi, MS 39533
(601) 435-1968 (hotline)

## Missouri

State agency: Missouri Commission
on Human Rights
P.O. Box 1129
Jefferson City, MO 65102
(314) 751-3325
(800) 877-6247

Women's Self Help Center
2838 Olive Street
St. Louis, MO 63103
(314) 531-9100 (office)
(314) 531-2003 (twenty-four-hour
hotline)
Offers counseling, referrals

YWCA Women's Resource Center
140 North Brentwood Avenue
Clayton, MO 63105
(314) 726-6665
Offers counseling, legal referrals

## Montana

State agency: Montana Human Rights
Commission
616 Helena Avenue, Suite 302
P.O. Box 1728
Helena, MT 59624-1728
(406) 444-2884
(800) 542-0807

Women's Place
501 West Alder
Missoula, MT 59802
(406) 543-3320 (office)
(406) 543-7606 (twenty-four-hour
crisis hotline)
Offers counseling and legal referrals

## Nebraska

State agency: Nebraska Equal
Employment Opportunity
Commission
301 Centennial Mall South
5th Floor
P.O. Box 94934
Lincoln, NE 68509
(402) 471-2024

University of Nebraska Women's
Center
117 Nebraska Union
Lincoln, NE 68588-0446
(402) 472-2597

Women Against Violence
(402) 345-7273

## Nevada

State agency: Nevada Equal Rights
Commission
1515 Tropicana Avenue, Suite 590
Las Vegas, NV 89158
(702) 486-7161 (Las Vegas)
(702) 688-1288 (Reno)

Crisis Call Center
P.O. Box 8016
Reno, NV 89507
(702) 323-4533 (office)
Makes legal referrals

## New Hampshire

State agency: New Hampshire
Commission for Human Rights
163 Loudon Road
Concord, NH 03301-6053
(603) 271-2767
Publishes the especially helpful "A
Manual on Sexual Harassment"

Sexual Assault Support Services
7 Junkins Avenue
Portsmouth, NH 03801
(603) 436-4107 (twenty-four-hour
hotline)
Offers legal referrals, education and
workshops, support groups

University of New Hampshire
Sexual Harassment and Rape
Prevention (SHARP)
Huddleston Hall
Durham, NH 03824
(603) 862-3494 (hotline, Mon.–Fri.,
8 A.M.–4:30 P.M.)
(603) 862-1212 (hotline, after
4:30 P.M.)
Offers counseling, support groups,
crisis and academic intervention, legal
assistance, and community outreach
including to high schools

## New Jersey

State agency: New Jersey Division on
Civil Rights
383 West State Street
Trenton, NJ 08618
(609) 292-4605

New Jersey Coalition Against Sexual
Assault
(908) 418-1354
Offers counseling, information

Rutgers Law School
Women's Rights Litigation Clinic
15 Washington Street
Newark, NJ 07102
(201) 648-5637
Offers information and litigation
about harassment

YWCA
140 East Hanover Street
Trenton, NJ 08608
(609) 989-9592 (office)
(609) 989-9332 (hotline)
Offers counseling, information,
referrals

**New Mexico**

State agency: New Mexico Human
Rights Commission
Aspen Plaza
1596 Pacheco Street
Santa Fe, NM 87501
(505) 827-6838

Rape Crisis Center
1025 Hermosa, S.E.
Albuquerque, NM 87108
(505) 266-7711 (hotline)

**New York**

State agency: New York State
Division of Human Rights
Office of Sexual Harassment Issues
55 Hanson Place, Suite 346
Brooklyn, NY 11217
(718) 722-2060
(800) 427-2773

Jefferson County Women's Center
120 Arcade Street
Watertown, NY 13601
(315) 782-1855
Offers counseling, support groups,
education on sexual harassment for
schools and businesses

New York Asian Women's Center
39 Bowery, Box 375
New York, NY 10002
(212) 732-5230
Offers counseling, legal, and other
referrals

9 to 5: National Organization of
Working Women
63 Jerusalem Avenue
Hempstead, NY 11550
(516) 485-6787
Offers counseling, legal, and other
referrals

NOW–NYC Hotline
15 West 18th Street
New York, NY 10011
(212) 989-7230

**North Carolina**

State agency (for private employees):
North Carolina Human Relations
Commission
121 West Jones Street
Raleigh, NC 27603
(919) 733-7996
(800) 699-4000

State agency (for public employees):
North Carolina State Office of
Administrative Hearings
424 North Blount Street
Raleigh, NC 27601
(919) 733-2691

North Carolina Equity
505 Oberlin Road
Raleigh, NC 27605
(919) 833-4055 (office)
(800) 451-8065 (hotline)

North Carolina Council for Women
James K. Polk Building
500 West Trade Building, Box 360
Charlotte, NC 28202
(704) 342-6367 (Charlotte)
(910) 334-5094 (Greensboro)
(704) 251-6169 (Asheville)
(919) 514-4869 (New Bern)
(919) 830-6595 (Greenville)

## North Dakota

State agency: North Dakota
Department of Labor
State Capitol Building
600 East Boulevard
Bismarck, ND 58505
(701) 328-2660

University of North Dakota
Women's Center
305 Hamline Street
Grand Forks, ND 58203
(701) 777-4300

## Ohio

State agency: Ohio Civil Rights
Commission
220 Parsons Avenue
Columbus, OH 43215
(216) 379-3100 (Akron)
(513) 852-3344 (Cincinnati)
(216) 787-3150 (Cleveland)
(614) 466-5928 (Columbus)
(513) 285-6500 (Dayton)
(419) 245-2900 (Toledo)

Committee Against Sexual Harassment
(CASH)
c/o YWCA
65 South 4th Street
Columbus, OH 43215
(614) 224-9121
Offers advice and referrals

Lorain County Rape Crisis Center
W. G. Nord Community Health
Center
6140 South Broadway
Lorain, OH 44053
(216) 233-7273 (office)
(800) 888-6161 (twenty-four-hour
hotline)
Offers support, legal and counseling
referrals, education

9 to 5: National Organization of
Working Women
614 Superior Avenue, N.W.
Cleveland, OH 44113
(216) 566-9308 (office)
(216) 621-9449
Makes referrals to counselors,
attorneys, support groups

Victims Advocacy Program, The Link
315 Thurston Avenue
Bowling Green, OH 43402
(419) 352-5387 (office)
(800) 472-9411 (hotline)
Offers support and legal referrals

YWCA Rape Crisis Center
1018 Jefferson
Toledo, OH 43624
(419) 241-7006 (office)
(419) 241-7273 (twenty-four-hour
hotline)
Offers counseling, legal referrals

## Oklahoma

State agency: Oklahoma Human
Rights Commission
2101 North Lincoln Boulevard
Room 480
Oklahoma City, OK 73105
(405) 521-3441 (Oklahoma City)
(918) 581-2733 (Tulsa)

Call Rape
2121 South Columbia, Room LL6
Tulsa, OK 74114
(918) 744-7273 (twenty-four-hour
crisis line)
Offers counseling, support groups,
legal referrals

## Oregon

State agency: Oregon Bureau of Labor
and Industry—Civil Rights Division
Suite 1070
800 Northeast Oregon Street, no. 32
Portland, OR 97232
(503) 731-4075, ext. 421 (Portland)
(503) 687-7460 (Eugene)

Columbia County Women's Resource
Center
Good Samaritan Medical Mall
Route 30
P.O. Box 22
St. Helens, OR 97051
(503) 397-0578 (office)
(503) 397-6161 (hotline)
Offers support, referrals

Portland Women's Crisis Line
P.O. Box 42610
Portland, OR 97242
(503) 232-9751 (office)
(503) 235-5333 (twenty-four-hour
hotline)

Sexual Assault Support Services
630 Lincoln Street
Eugene, OR 97401
(503) 484-9791 (office)
(800) 788-4247 (hotline)
Offers telephone support, legal
referrals

Women's Crisis Center
P.O. Box 187
Tillamook, OR 97141
(305) 842-9486 (twenty-four-hour
hotline)
Offers counseling, legal referrals,
community education

## Pennsylvania

State agency: Pennsylvania Human
Relations Commission
101 South Second Street, Suite 300
Harrisburg, PA 17105-3145
(717) 787-9784 (Harrisburg)
(215) 560-2496 (Philadelphia)
(412) 565-5395 (Pittsburgh)

Philadelphia Commission on Human
Relations
34 South 11th Street, 6th Floor
Philadelphia, PA 19107-3654
(215) 686-4692
Files complaints (for city of
Philadelphia only)

Women's Alliance for Job Equity
(WAJE)
1422 Chestnut Street, Suite 1100
Philadelphia, PA 19102
(215) 561-1873
Offers support groups, training,
education, and advocacy

Women's Law Project
125 South Ninth Street, Suite 401
Philadelphia, PA 19107
(215) 928-9801
Makes referrals

## Rhode Island

State agency: Rhode Island
Commission for Human Rights
10 Abbot Park Place
Providence, RI 02903
(401) 277-2661

Brown University
Sara Doyle Women's Center
(401) 863-2189
Offers information, referrals

Rape Crisis Center
300 Richmond Street, Suite 205
Providence, RI 02903
(401) 421-4100 (hotline)

## South Carolina

State agency: South Carolina Human
Affairs Commission
2611 Forest Drive
P.O. Box 4490
Columbia, SC 29240
(803) 253-6339
(800) 521-0725

Crisisline
(803) 271-8888
Offers information, referrals

My Sister's House
P.O. Box 5341
North Charleston, SC 29406
(803) 747-4069 (office)
(800) 273-4673 (twenty-four-hour
hotline)
Offers support groups, legal referrals,
education

## South Dakota

State agency: South Dakota Division
of Human Rights
222 East Capitol, Suite 11
Pierre, SD 57501-5070
(605) 773-4493

Citizens Against Rape and Domestic
Violence
300 North Dakota Avenue, Suite 220
Sioux Falls, SD 57102
(605) 339-0116
Offers information, legal and
counseling referrals

Volunteer and Information Center
(800) 339-4537

## Tennessee

State agency: Tennessee Human
Rights Commission
530 Church Street, Suite 400
Nashville, TN 37243
(615) 741-5825

Family Services of Memphis
2400 Poplar Avenue, Suite 500
Memphis, TN 38112
(901) 324-3637 (office)
(901) 274-7477 (hotline)

## Texas

State agency: Texas Commission on
Human Rights
8100 Cameron Road, Building B
Suite 525
Austin, TX 78754
(512) 837-8534

The Dallas Rainbow Now Sexual
Harassment Support Group
608 Whistler
Arlington, TX 76006
(817) 792-3736
Offers support group; makes therapist
and attorney referrals

Texas Bar Referral, Legal Aid
205 West 9th Street, Suite 200
Austin, TX 78701
(800) 204-2222, x2146 (Texas Bar)
(512) 476-7244 (Legal Aid)

Texas Civil Rights Project
(512) 474-5073
Offers information and referrals

University YWCA
Women's Counseling and Resource
Center
55 North IH35, Suite 230
Austin, TX 78702
Offers counseling, referrals

Women's Counseling and Resource
Center
(512) 472-3053

## Utah

State agency: Utah Industrial
Commission
Anti-Discrimination Division
160 East 300 South
Salt Lake City, UT 84114
(801) 530-6801

Utah Women's Lobby
P.O. Box 1586
Salt Lake City, UT 84110-1586

## Vermont

State agency: Vermont Attorney
General's Office
Civil Rights Division
109 State Street
Montpelier, VT 05609
(802) 828-3657

Those Who Mourn
P.O. Box 937
Wilder, VT 05088
(802) 296-7109

## Virginia

State agency: Council on Human
Rights
1100 Bank Street
Washington Building, 12th Floor
Richmond, VA 23219
(804) 225-2292

Sexual Assault Resource Agency
(SARA)
P.O. Box 6705
Charlottesville, VA 22906
(804) 295-7273 (office)
(804) 977-7273 (hotline)


## Washington

State agency: Washington State
Human Rights Commission
711 South Capitol Way, Suite 402
Olympia, WA 98504
(360) 753-6770 (Olympia)
(206) 464-6500 (Seattle)
(509) 456-4473 (Spokane)
(509) 575-2772 (Yakima)


Northwest Women's Law Center
119 South Main Street
Suite 330
Seattle, WA 98104
(206) 621-7691
Offers information and attorney
referrals


## West Virginia

State agency: West Virginia Human
Rights Commission
1321 Plaza East, Room 106
Charleston, WV 25301-1400
(304) 348-2616


Rape and Domestic Violence
Information Center
104 East High Street
Kingwood, WV 26537
(304) 329-1687


Women and Employment, Inc.
(304) 345-1298


## Wisconsin

State agency: Wisconsin Department
of Industry, Labor and Human
Relations
Equal Rights Division
P.O. Box 8928
201 East Washington Avenue
Madison, WI 53708
(608) 266-7552


Counseling Center of Milwaukee
Milwaukee, WI
(414) 271-2565
Offers counseling, legal referrals


9 to 5: National Association of
Working Women
Milwaukee, WI 53203
(414) 272-7795
Offers phone counseling, legal
referrals


## Wyoming

State agency: Wyoming Fair
Employment Commission
6101 Yellowstone, Room 259C
Cheyenne, WY 82002
(307) 777-7261


Women's Center Collective
P.O. Box 581
Sheridan, WY 82801
(307) 672-7471 (office)
(307) 672-3222 (hotline)
Offers counseling, information

# APPENDIX B
## EEOC FIELD OFFICES
## (IN ALPHABETICAL ORDER BY CITY)

505 Marquette N.W., Suite 900
Albuquerque, NM 87102
(505) 766-2061

75 Piedmont Avenue N.E.
Suite 1100
Atlanta, GA 30335
(404) 331-6093

111 Market Place, Suite 4000
Baltimore, MD 21202
(301) 962-3932

1900 Third Avenue North, Suite 101
Birmingham, AL 35203
(205) 731-0082

1 Congress Street, Room 100
10th Floor
Boston, MA 02114
(617) 565-3200

28 Church Street, Room 301
Buffalo, NY 14202
(716) 846-4441

5500 Central Avenue
Charlotte, NC 28212
(704) 567-7100

536 South Clark Street, Room 930A
Chicago, IL 60605
(312) 353-2713

525 Vine Street, Suite 810
Cincinnati, OH 45202
(513) 684-2851

1375 Euclid Avenue, Room 600
Cleveland, OH 44115
(216) 522-2001

8303 Elmbrook Drive
Dallas, TX 75247
(214) 767-7015

1845 Sherman Street, 2d Floor
Denver, CO 80203
(303) 866-1300

477 Michigan Avenue, Room 1540
Detroit, MI 48226
(313) 226-7636


The Commons, Building C, Suite 100
El Paso, TX 79902
(915) 534-6550


1313 P Street, Suite 103
Fresno, CA 93721
(209) 487-5793


324 West Market Street, Room B27
Greensboro, NC 27402
(919) 333-5174


15 South Main Street, Suite 530
Greenville, SC 29601
(803) 241-4400


677 Ala Moana Boulevard, Suite 404
Honolulu, HI 96813
(808) 541-3120


1919 Smith Street, 7th Floor
Houston, TX 77002
(713) 653-3377


46 East Ohio Street, Room 456
Indianapolis, IN 46204
(317) 226-7212


207 West Amite Street
Jackson, MS 39269
(601) 965-4537


911 Walnut, 10th Floor
Kansas City, MO 64106
(816) 426-5773


320 West Capitol Avenue, Suite 621
Little Rock, AR 72201
(501) 324-5060


3660 Wilshire Boulevard, 5th Floor
Los Angeles, CA 90010
(213) 251-7278


600 Martin Luther King, Jr., Place
Suite 268
Louisville, KY 40202
(502) 582-6082


1407 Union Avenue, Suite 621
Memphis, TN 38104
(901) 722-2617


1 Northeast First Street, 6th Floor
Miami, FL 33132
(305) 536-4491


310 West Wisconsin Avenue
Suite 800
Milwaukee, WI 53203
(414) 297-1111


220 Second Street South, Room 108
Minneapolis, MN 55401
(612) 370-3330


50 Vantage Way, Suite 202
Nashville, TN 37228
(615) 736-5820


60 Park Place, Room 301
Newark, NJ 07102
(201) 645-6383


701 Loyola Avenue, Suite 600
New Orleans, LA 70113
(504) 589-2329

90 Church Street, Room 1501
New York, NY 10007
(212) 264-7161

252 Monticello Avenue
SMA Building, 1st Floor
Norfolk, VA 23510
(804) 441-3470

1333 Broadway, Room 430
Oakland, CA 94612
(510) 273-7588

531 Couch Drive
Oklahoma City, OK 94612
(405) 231-4911

1421 Cherry Street, 10th Floor
Philadelphia, PA 19102
(215) 656-7020

4520 North Central Avenue
Suite 300
Phoenix, AZ 85012
(602) 640-5000

1000 Liberty Avenue, Room 2038A
Pittsburgh, PA 15222
(412) 644-3444

1309 Annapolis Drive
Raleigh, NC 27601
(919) 856-4064

3600 West Broad Street, 2d Floor
Richmond, VA 23230
(804) 771-2692

5410 Fredericksburg Road, Suite 200
San Antonio, TX 78229
(512) 229-4810

401 B Street, Suite 1550
San Diego, CA 92101
(619) 557-7235

901 Market Street, Suite 500
San Francisco, CA 94103
(415) 744-6500

96 North Third Street
San Jose, CA 95113
(408) 291-7352

10 Whitaker Street, Suite B
Savannah, GA 31401
(912) 944-4234

2815 Second Avenue, Suite 500
Seattle, WA 98121
(206) 553-0968

625 North Euclid Street, 5th Floor
St. Louis, MO 63108
(314) 425-6585

501 East Polk Street, 10th Floor
Tampa, FL 33602
(813) 228-2310

1400 L Street, N.W., 2d Floor
Washington, DC 20005
(202) 275-7377

# APPENDIX C
# SAMPLE SEXUAL HARASSMENT POLICY

*I thank the Indiana Civil Rights Commission, the Kansas Commission on Human Rights, the Montana Human Rights Division of the Department of Labor and Industry, and the New Hampshire Commission for Human Rights for their very helpful brochures and model sexual harassment policies, upon which I have drawn in composing the document that follows.*

**Statement of Philosophy**     Sexual harassment of employees, customers, and any other individual is prohibited and will not be tolerated. It is a goal of [name of company or organization] to create a workplace and a working [or learning] environment that promotes equal opportunity and prohibits discriminatory practices, including sexual harassment. It is the policy of this organization to provide all of its employees [students] with a work [or learning] environment that is as free of unlawful discrimination and harassment as possible.

Harassment of employees by co-workers, faculty, peers, supervisors, managers, customers, or vendors will not be permitted, regardless of their working relationship. Reprisals for reporting harassment are also prohibited. Harassment and reprisals for reporting harassment are serious violations of this organization's work rules and will be subject to discipline up to and including termination.

**Definition**     Sexual harassment includes unwelcome verbal or physical conduct of a sexual nature when:

Submission to the conduct is implicitly or explicitly made a term or condition of employment;

Submission to or rejection of the conduct is used as the basis for an employment decision affecting the individual;

or

The conduct has the purpose or effect of unreasonably interfering with an individual's work performance or creating an intimidating, offensive, or hostile working environment.

Examples of prohibited sexual harassment include, but are not limited to:

Sexual innuendo, suggestive comments, insults, threats, jokes;

Suggestive or insulting noises, staring, leering, whistling, or making obscene gestures;

Propositions or pressure to engage in sexual activity;

Sexual assault or coercing sexual intercourse;

Touching, pinching, cornering, or brushing the body;

Inappropriate comments concerning appearance;

Sexual or sexually insulting written communications, or public postings, including in electronic media;

Display of magazines, books, or pictures with a sexual connotation;

A pattern of hiring or promoting sex partners over more qualified persons;

Any harassing behavior, whether or not sexual in nature, that is directed toward a person because of the person's gender, including, but not limited to, hazing employees working in nontraditional work environments.

**Nonretaliation**      This organization will not retaliate against any applicant, employee, or past employee for opposing sexual harassment, filing a harassment complaint, or testifying or participating in any other manner in a harassment investigation or proceeding.

**Grievance Procedure**      Individuals who believe that they or others have been subjected to harassment from a co-worker, supervisor, manager, customer, or vendor can report the conduct to their supervisor, manager, [human resources or other sexual harassment officer], or others designated within the organization. Their names and telephone numbers are: [                    ]. While employees are encouraged to report instances of harassment to their supervisors and managers first, they are not required to do so, and they may instead contact employee assistance for counseling, [other resources the organization may suggest], [the state agency], or the U.S. Equal Employment Opportunity Commission.

**Investigations**      Investigations must be handled in as timely and confidential a manner as possible. Any supervisor, manager, or other person of responsibility within the organization shall, upon either observing or receiving reports of sexual harassment, immediately notify the organization's sexual harassment officer [or chief executive], who will arrange a fair and thorough investigation of the complaint, and make a factual report no later than ten working days after receiving notice of the alleged violation. The investigation shall include, but not necessarily be limited to, interviewing as many individuals as possible who have knowledge of the matter and reviewing any relevant documents.

Employees named in harassment complaints will be given sufficient information about the allegation to provide them a reasonable opportunity to respond before any corrective action or discipline is imposed. Named employees should not be assumed to have violated this policy unless and until the investigation establishes that they have done so.

Upon receipt of a complaint alleging sexual harassment, [the organization] shall take all appropriate steps to prevent the alleged conduct from continuing pending completion of the investigation. [The organization] will determine the steps to be taken by balancing the rights of the alleged victim, including the severity of the alleged conduct, and the rights of the alleged harasser.

Within two working days of receiving the factual report, [the chief executive of the organization] will, in writing, inform the complainant, any other employees directly involved, their immediate supervisors, and the sexual harassment officer of the results of the investigation, including whether or not a finding of violating this sexual harassment policy was made. Otherwise, the factual report and the decision shall remain confidential and shall be disseminated only to persons having a need or right to know that outweighs the privacy rights of the individuals involved.

If the results of the investigation establish that there is insufficient evidence that a policy violation occurred, [the organization] will inform all parties involved that the matter is concluded. If the results of the investigation establish that a policy violation occurred, [the organization] will take appropriate disciplinary action, up to and including termination of employment. Where the investigation establishes a violation of the policy that does not result in termination, [the organization] is responsible for carefully explaining this policy to the harasser, suggesting ways to correct the behavior, and informing him or her that any further instances of harassment may result in immediate termination of employment.

# APPENDIX D
# COURT OPINIONS

*ELLISON V. BRADY*

## UNITED STATES COURT OF APPEALS, NINTH CIRCUIT

---------------

No. 89-15248

---------------

KERRY ELLISON, PLAINTIFF-APPELLANT V. NICHOLAS F. BRADY,* SECRETARY OF THE TREASURY, DEFENDANT-APPELLEE.

**Argued and Submitted April 19, 1990.**
**Decided Jan. 23, 1991.**
**Dissent Amended Feb. 5, 1991.**
**Appeal from the United States District Court for the Northern District of California.**
**Before Beezer and Kozinski, Circuit Judges, and Stephens,** District Judge.*

Beezer, Circuit Judge:

Kerry Ellison appeals the district court's order granting summary judgment to the Secretary of the Treasury on her sexual harassment action brought under Title VII of the Civil Rights Act of 1964. 42 U.S.C. § 2000e (1982). This appeal presents two important issues: (1) what test should be applied to determine

---

* Nicholas F. Brady is substituted for James A. Baker III as Secretary of the Treasury, pursuant to Rule 43(c)(1) of the Federal Rules of Appellate Procedure.
** The Honorable Albert Lee Stephens, Senior United States District Judge for the Central District of California, sitting by designation.

whether conduct is sufficiently severe or pervasive to alter the conditions of employment and create a hostile working environment, and (2) what remedial actions can shield employers from liability for sexual harassment by co-workers. The district court held that Ellison did not state a prima facie case of hostile environment sexual harassment. We reverse and remand.

Both issues require a detailed analysis of the facts, which we consider in the light most favorable to Ellison, the non moving party. *Sierra Club v. Penfold*, 857 F.2d 1307, 1320 (9th Cir.1988). We review summary judgments de novo. *Id.*

I

Kerry Ellison worked as a revenue agent for the Internal Revenue Service in San Mateo, California. During her initial training in 1984 she met Sterling Gray, another trainee, who was also assigned to the San Mateo office. The two co-workers never became friends, and they did not work closely together.

Gray's desk was twenty feet from Ellison's desk, two rows behind and one row over. Revenue agents in the San Mateo office often went to lunch in groups. In June of 1986 when no one else was in the office, Gray asked Ellison to lunch. She accepted. Gray had to pick up his son's forgotten lunch, so they stopped by Gray's house. He gave Ellison a tour of his house.

Ellison alleges that after the June lunch Gray started to pester her with unnecessary questions and hang around her desk. On October 9, 1986, Gray asked Ellison out for a drink after work. She declined, but she suggested that they have lunch the following week. She did not want to have lunch alone with him, and she tried to stay away from the office during lunch time. One day during the following week, Gray uncharacteristically dressed in a three-piece suit and asked Ellison out for lunch. Again, she did not accept.

On October 22, 1986, Gray handed Ellison a note he wrote on a telephone message slip which read:

> I cried over you last night and I'm totally drained today. I have never been in such constant term oil [sic]. Thank you for talking with me. I could not stand to feel your hatred for another day.

When Ellison realized that Gray wrote the note, she became shocked and frightened and left the room. Gray followed her into the hallway and demanded that she talk to him, but she left the building.

Ellison later showed the note to Bonnie Miller, who supervised both Ellison and Gray. Miller said "this is sexual harassment." Ellison asked Miller not to do anything about it. She wanted to try to handle it herself. Ellison asked a male co-worker to talk to Gray, to tell him that she was not interested in him and to leave her alone. The next day, Thursday, Gray called in sick.

Ellison did not work on Friday, and on the following Monday, she started four weeks of training in St. Louis, Missouri. Gray mailed her a card and a typed, single-spaced, three-page letter. She describes this letter as "twenty times, a hundred times weirder" than the prior note. Gray wrote, in part:

> I know that you are worth knowing with or without sex. . . . Leaving aside the hassles and disasters of recent weeks. I have enjoyed you so much over these past few months. Watching you. Experiencing you from O so far away. Admiring your style and elan. . . . Don't you think it odd that two people who have never even talked together, alone, are striking off such intense sparks. . . . I will [write] another letter in the near future.[1]

Explaining her reaction, Ellison stated: "I just thought he was crazy. I thought he was nuts. I didn't know what he would do next. I was frightened."

She immediately telephoned Miller. Ellison told her supervisor that she was frightened and really upset. She requested that Miller transfer either her or Gray because she would not be comfortable working in the same office with him. Miller asked Ellison to send a copy of the card and letter to San Mateo.

Miller then telephoned her supervisor, Joe Benton, and discussed the problem. That same day she had a counseling session with Gray. She informed him that he was entitled to union representation. During this meeting, she told Gray to leave Ellison alone.

At Benton's request, Miller apprised the labor relations department of the situation. She also reminded Gray many times over the next few weeks that he must not contact Ellison in any way. Gray subsequently transferred to the San Francisco office on November 24, 1986. Ellison returned from St. Louis in late November and did not discuss the matter further with Miller.

After three weeks in San Francisco, Gray filed union grievances requesting a return to the San Mateo office. The IRS and the union settled the grievances in Gray's favor, agreeing to allow him to transfer back to the San Mateo office provided that he spend four more months in San Francisco and promise not to bother Ellison. On January 28, 1987, Ellison first learned of Gray's request in a letter from Miller explaining that Gray would return to the San Mateo office. The letter indicated that management decided to resolve Ellison's problem with a six-month separation, and that it would take additional action if the problem recurred.

After receiving the letter, Ellison was "frantic." She filed a formal complaint

---

1. In the middle of the long letter Gray did say "I am obligated to you so much that if you want me to leave you alone I will. . . . If you want me to forget you entirely, I can not do that."

alleging sexual harassment on January 30, 1987, with the IRS. She also obtained permission to transfer to San Francisco temporarily when Gray returned.

Gray sought joint counseling. He wrote Ellison another letter which still sought to maintain the idea that he and Ellison had some type of relationship.[2]

The IRS employee investigating the allegation agreed with Ellison's supervisor that Gray's conduct constituted sexual harassment. In its final decision, however, the Treasury Department rejected Ellison's complaint because it believed that the complaint did not describe a pattern or practice of sexual harassment covered by the EEOC regulations. After an appeal, the EEOC affirmed the Treasury Department's decision on a different ground. It concluded that the agency took adequate action to prevent the repetition of Gray's conduct.

Ellison filed a complaint in September of 1987 in federal district court. The court granted the government's motion for summary judgment on the ground that Ellison had failed to state a prima facie case of sexual harassment due to a hostile working environment. Ellison appeals.

## II

Congress added the word "sex" to Title VII of the Civil Rights Act of 1964[3] at the last minute on the floor of the House of Representatives. 110 Cong.Rec. 2,577–2,584 (1964). Virtually no legislative history provides guidance to courts interpreting the prohibition of sex discrimination. In *Meritor Savings Bank v. Vinson*, 477 U.S. 57, 106 S.Ct. 2399, 91 L.Ed.2d 49 (1986), the Supreme Court held that sexual harassment constitutes sex discrimination in violation of Title VII.

Courts have recognized different forms of sexual harassment. In "quid pro quo" cases, employers condition employment benefits on sexual favors. In "hostile environment" cases, employees work in offensive or abusive environments.[4] A. Larson, *Employment Discrimination* § 41.61 at 8–151 (1989). This case, like *Meritor*, involves a hostile environment claim.

The Supreme Court in *Meritor* held that Mechelle Vinson's working conditions constituted a hostile environment in violation of Title VII's prohibition of sex discrimination. Vinson's supervisor made repeated demands for sexual favors, usually at work, both during and after business hours. Vinson initially refused her

---

2. It is unclear from the record on appeal whether Ellison received the third letter.

3. That statute makes it "an unlawful employment practice for an employer . . . to discriminate against any individual with respect to his compensation, terms, conditions, or privileges of employment, because of such individual's race, color, religion, sex, or national origin." 42 U.S.C. § 2000e-2(a)(1) (1982).

4. Some courts have entertained causes of action for sexual harassment which do not fall squarely within the quid pro quo cases or the hostile environment cases. For example, some courts have classified harassment based on the victim's gender as sexual harassment where the conduct or language is not sexual in nature. *See, e.g., Hall v. Gus Construction Co.*, 842 F.2d 1010, 1014 (8th Cir.1988). Our examples are illustrative and not exclusive because we realize that sexual harassment is a rapidly expanding area of the law.

employer's sexual advances, but eventually acceded because she feared losing her job. They had intercourse over forty times. She additionally testified that he "fondled her in front of other employees, followed her into the women's restroom when she went there alone, exposed himself to her, and even forcibly raped her on several occasions." *Meritor,* 477 U.S. at 60, 106 S.Ct. at 2402. The Court had no difficulty finding this environment hostile. *Id.* at 67, 106 S.Ct. at 2405–06.

[1] Since *Meritor,* we have not often reached the merits of a hostile environment sexual harassment claim. In *Jordan v. Clark,* 847 F.2d 1368, 1373 (9th Cir.1988), *cert. denied sub nom., Jordan v. Hodel,* 488 U.S. 1006, 109 S.Ct. 786, 102 L.Ed.2d 778 (1989), we explained that a hostile environment exists when an employee can show (1) that he or she was subjected to sexual advances, requests for sexual favors, or other verbal or physical conduct of a sexual nature,[5](2) that this conduct was unwelcome, and (3) that the conduct was sufficiently severe or pervasive to alter the conditions of the victim's employment and create an abusive working environment.

[2] In *Jordan,* we reviewed for clear error the district court's determination that an employee was not subjected to particular unwelcome advances. *Id.* at 1375. We explained that we will review de novo a district court's final conclusion that conduct is not severe enough or pervasive enough to constitute an abusive environment. *Id.* at n. 7. We affirmed the district court's judgment in *Jordan* because we did not find its factual findings clearly erroneous. *Id. See also Vasconcelos v. Meese,* 907 F.2d 111, 112 (9th Cir.1990) (affirming district court's decision that the working environment was not sexually hostile because the district court's factual findings were not clearly erroneous).

We had another opportunity to examine a hostile working environment claim of sexual harassment in *E.E.O.C. v. Hacienda Hotel,* 881 F.2d 1504 (9th Cir.1989). In that case the district court found a hostile working environment where the hotel's male chief of engineering frequently made sexual comments and sexual advances to the maids, and where a female supervisor called her female employees "dog[s]" and "whore[s]." *Id.* at 1508. Upon a de novo review of the facts found by the district court, we agreed that the conduct was sufficiently severe and pervasive to alter the conditions of employment and create a hostile working environment.

III

The parties ask us to determine if Gray's conduct, as alleged by Ellison, was sufficiently severe or pervasive to alter the conditions of Ellison's employment and

---

5. Here, the government argues that Gray's conduct was not of a sexual nature. The three-page letter, however, makes several references to sex and constitutes verbal conduct of a sexual nature. We need not and do not decide whether a party can state a cause of action for a sexually discriminatory working environment under Title VII when the conduct in question is not sexual. *See Andrews v. City of Philadelphia,* 895 F.2d 1469, 1485 (3rd Cir.1990) (conduct need not be sexual); *Hall v. Gus Construction Co.,* 842 F.2d 1010, 1014 (8th Cir.1988) (conduct need not be sexual).

create an abusive working environment. The district court, with little Ninth Circuit case law to look to for guidance, held that Ellison did not state a prima facie case of sexual harassment due to a hostile working environment. It believed that Gray's conduct was "isolated and genuinely trivial." We disagree.

We begin our analysis of the third part of the framework we set forth in *Jordan* with a closer look at *Meritor*. The Supreme Court in *Meritor* explained that courts may properly look to guidelines issued by the Equal Employment Opportunity Commission (EEOC) for guidance when examining hostile environment claims of sexual harassment. 477 U.S. at 65, 106 S.Ct. at 2404–05. The EEOC guidelines describe hostile environment harassment as "conduct [which] has the purpose or effect of unreasonably interfering with an individual's work performance or creating an intimidating, hostile, or offensive working environment." 29 C.F.R. § 1604.11(a)(3). The EEOC, in accord with a substantial body of judicial decisions, has concluded that "Title VII affords employees the right to work in an environment free from discriminatory intimidation, ridicule, and insult." 477 U.S. at 65, 106 S.Ct. at 2405.

The Supreme Court cautioned, however, that not all harassment affects a "term, condition, or privilege" of employment within the meaning of Title VII. For example, the "mere utterance of an ethnic or racial epithet which engenders offensive feelings in an employee" is not, by itself, actionable under Title VII. *Id.* at 67, 106 S.Ct. at 2405. To state a claim under Title VII, sexual harassment "must be sufficiently severe or pervasive to alter the conditions of the victim's employment and create an abusive working environment." *Id.*

[3] The Supreme Court drew its limiting language from *Rogers v. E.E.O.C.*, 454 F.2d 234 (5th Cir.1971), *cert. denied*, 406 U.S. 957, 92 S.Ct. 2058, 32 L.Ed.2d 343 (1972), the first case to recognize a hostile racial environment claim under Title VII. The *Rogers* phrasing limits hostile environment claims to cases where conduct alters the conditions of employment and creates an abusive working environment. The EEOC guidelines, drawing upon *Rogers* and other decisions, indicate that sexual harassment violates Title VII where conduct creates an intimidating, hostile, or offensive environment *or* where it unreasonably interferes with work performance. 29 C.F.R. § 1604.11(a)(3).

We do not think that these standards are inconsistent. The Supreme Court used the words "abusive" and "hostile" synonymously in *Meritor*. 477 U.S. at 66, 106 S.Ct. at 2405. The *Meritor* Court also approved of and paid detailed attention to the EEOC's guidelines, and it implicitly adopted the EEOC's position that sexual harassment which unreasonably interferes with work performance violates Title VII. Similarly, although we only expressly incorporated the limiting language from *Rogers* in the third part of our framework in *Jordan*, that part also encompasses the EEOC's requirements in 29 C.F.R. § 1604.11(a)(3). Conduct which unreasonably interferes with work performance can alter a condition of employment and create an abusive working environment. *Contra* Pollack, *Sexual Harassment: Women's*

*Experience vs. Legal Definitions,* 13 Harv. Women's Law J. 35, 60 (1990) (arguing that the *Meritor* court opted for the strict standard enunciated in *Rogers* instead of the more lenient EEOC standard).

Although *Meritor* and our previous cases establish the framework for the resolution of hostile environment cases, they do not dictate the outcome of this case. Gray's conduct falls somewhere between forcible rape and the mere utterance of an epithet. 477 U.S. at 60, 67, 106 S.Ct. at 2402, 2405–06. His conduct was not as pervasive as the sexual comments and sexual advances in *Hacienda Hotel,* which we held created an unlawfully hostile working environment. 881 F.2d 1504.

The government asks us to apply the reasoning of other courts which have declined to find Title VII violations on more egregious facts. In *Scott v. Sears, Roebuck & Co.,* 798 F.2d 210, 212 (7th Cir.1986), the Seventh Circuit analyzed a female employee's working conditions for sexual harassment. It noted that she was repeatedly propositioned and winked at by her supervisor. When she asked for assistance, he asked "what will I get for it?" Co-workers slapped her buttocks and commented that she must moan and groan during sex. The court examined the evidence to see if "the demeaning conduct and sexual stereotyping cause[d] such anxiety and debilitation to the plaintiff that working conditions were 'poisoned' within the meaning of Title VII." *Id.* at 213. The court did not consider the environment sufficiently hostile. *Id.* at 214.

Similarly, in *Rabidue v. Osceola Refining Co.,* 805 F.2d 611 (6th Cir.1986), *cert. denied,* 481 U.S. 1041, 107 S.Ct. 1983, 95 L.Ed.2d 823 (1987), the Sixth Circuit refused to find a hostile environment where the workplace contained posters of naked and partially dressed women, and where a male employee customarily called women "whores," "cunt," "pussy," and "tits," referred to plaintiff as "fat ass," and specifically stated, "All that bitch needs is a good lay." Over a strong dissent, the majority held that the sexist remarks and the pin-up posters had only a de minimis effect and did not seriously affect the plaintiff's psychological well-being.

We do not agree with the standards set forth in *Scott and Rabidue,*[6] and we choose not to follow those decisions.[7] Neither *Scott*'s search for "anxiety and debilitation" sufficient to "poison" a working environment nor *Rabidue*'s requirement that a plaintiff's psychological well-being be "seriously affected" follows directly from

---

6. We note that the Sixth Circuit has called *Rabidue* into question in at least two subsequent opinions. In *Yates v. Avco Corp.,* 819 F.2d 630, 637 (6th Cir.1987), a panel of the Sixth Circuit expressly adopted one of the main arguments in the *Rabidue* dissent, that sexual harassment actions should be viewed from the victim's perspective. In *Davis v. Monsanto Chemical Co.,* 858 F.2d 345, 350 (6th Cir.1988), *cert. denied,* 490 U.S. 1110, 109 S.Ct. 3166, 104 L.Ed.2d 1028 (1989), the Sixth Circuit once again criticized *Rabidue*'s limited reading of Title VII. *See also Andrews v. City of Philadelphia,* 895 F.2d 1469, 1485 (3d Cir.1990) (explicitly rejecting *Rabidue* and holding that derogatory language directed at women and pornographic pictures of women serve as evidence of a hostile working environment).

7. We note that unlike this case, the plaintiffs in *Scott* and *Rabidue* alleged that a hostile working environment contributed to their discharge. We need not and do not address how or whether a discharge would alter our analysis.

language in *Meritor*.[8] It is the harasser's conduct which must be pervasive or severe, not the alteration in the conditions of employment. Surely, employees need not endure sexual harassment until their psychological well-being is seriously affected to the extent that they suffer anxiety and debilitation. *Accord, EEOC Policy Guidance on Sexual Harassment,* 8 Fair Employment Practices Manual (BNA) 405:6681, 6690, n. 20 (March 19, 1990). Although an isolated epithet by itself fails to support a cause of action for a hostile environment, Title VII's protection of employees from sex discrimination comes into play long before the point where victims of sexual harassment require psychiatric assistance.

[4] We have closely examined *Meritor* and our previous cases, and we believe that Gray's conduct was sufficiently severe and pervasive to alter the conditions of Ellison's employment and create an abusive working environment. We first note that the required showing of severity or seriousness of the harassing conduct varies inversely with the pervasiveness or frequency of the conduct. *See King v. Board of Regents of University of Wisconsin System,* 898 F.2d 533, 537 (7th Cir.1990) ("[a]lthough a single act can be enough, . . . generally, repeated incidents create a stronger claim of hostile environment, with the strength of the claim depending on the number of incidents and the intensity of each incident"). *Accord Andrews,* 895 F.2d at 1484; *Carrero v. New York City Housing Authority,* 890 F.2d 569, 578 (2d Cir.1989); EEOC Compliance Manual, § 615, ¶ 3112, C at 3243 (CCH 1988). For example, in *Vance v. Southern Bell Telephone and Telegraph Co.,* 863 F.2d 1503, 1510 (11th Cir.1989), the court held that two incidents in which a noose was found hung over an employee's work station were sufficiently severe to constitute a jury question on a racially hostile environment.

[5] Next, we believe that in evaluating the severity and pervasiveness of sexual harassment, we should focus on the perspective of the victim. *King,* 898 F.2d at 537; EEOC Compliance Manual (CCH) § 615, ¶ 3112, C at 3242 (1988) (courts "should consider the victim's perspective and not stereotyped notions of acceptable behavior"). If we only examined whether a reasonable person would engage in allegedly harassing conduct, we would run the risk of reinforcing the prevailing level of discrimination. Harassers could continue to harass merely because a particular discriminatory practice was common, and victims of harassment would have no remedy.

---

8. As we explained earlier, the Supreme Court in *Meritor* implicitly adopted the EEOC's position that sexual harassment which unreasonably interferes with work performance violates Title VII. 477 U.S. at 65, 106 S.Ct. at 2404–05. Conduct can unreasonably interfere with work performance without causing debilitation and without seriously affecting an employee's psychological well-being. Perhaps the confusion in *Scott* and *Rabidue* flows from a quotation in *Meritor* from *Rogers.* In its analysis, the *Rogers* court explained that "[o]ne can readily envision working environments so heavily polluted with discrimination as to destroy completely the emotional and psychological stability of minority group workers." *Meritor,* 477 U.S. at 66, 106 S.Ct. at 2405, *quoting Rogers,* 454 F.2d at 238. The *Rogers* court did *not* hold that a hostile environment only exists when the emotional and psychological stability of workers is completely destroyed.

We therefore prefer to analyze harassment from the victim's perspective. A complete understanding of the victim's view requires, among other things, an analysis of the different perspectives of men and women. Conduct that many men consider unobjectionable may offend many women. *See, e.g., Lipsett v. University of Puerto Rico,* 864 F.2d 881, 898 (1st Cir.1988) ("A male supervisor might believe, for example, that it is legitimate for him to tell a female subordinate that she has a 'great figure' or 'nice legs.' The female subordinate, however, may find such comments offensive"); *Yates,* 819 F.2d at 637, n. 2 ("men and women are vulnerable in different ways and offended by different behavior"). *See also* Ehrenreich, *Pluralist Myths and Powerless Men: The Ideology of Reasonableness in Sexual Harassment Law,* 99 Yale L.J. 1177, 1207–1208 (1990) (men tend to view some forms of sexual harassment as "harmless social interactions to which only overly-sensitive women would object"); Abrams, *Gender Discrimination and the Transformation of Workplace Norms,* 42 Vand.L.Rev. 1183, 1203 (1989) (the characteristically male view depicts sexual harassment as comparatively harmless amusement).

We realize that there is a broad range of viewpoints among women as a group, but we believe that many women share common concerns which men do not necessarily share.[9] For example, because women are disproportionately victims of rape and sexual assault, women have a stronger incentive to be concerned with sexual behavior.[10] Women who are victims of mild forms of sexual harassment may understandably worry whether a harasser's conduct is merely a prelude to violent sexual assault. Men, who are rarely victims of sexual assault, may view sexual conduct in a vacuum without a full appreciation of the social setting or the underlying threat of violence that a woman may perceive.

[6] In order to shield employers from having to accommodate the idiosyncratic concerns of the rare hyper-sensitive employee, we hold that a female plaintiff states a prima facie case of hostile environment sexual harassment when she alleges conduct which a reasonable woman[11] would consider sufficiently severe or pervasive to alter the conditions of employment and create an abusive working environ-

---

9. One writer explains: "While many women hold positive attitudes about uncoerced sex, their greater physical and social vulnerability to sexual coercion can make women wary of sexual encounters. Moreover, American women have been raised in a society where rape and sex-related violence have reached unprecedented levels, and a vast pornography industry creates continuous images of sexual coercion, objectification and violence. Finally, women as a group tend to hold more restrictive views of both the situation and type of relationship in which sexual conduct is appropriate. Because of the inequality and coercion with which it is so frequently associated in the minds of women, the appearance of sexuality in an unexpected context or a setting of ostensible equality can be an anguishing experience." Abrams, *Gender Discrimination and the Transformation of Workplace Norms,* 42 Vand.L.Rev. 1183, 1205 (1989).

10. United States Department of Justice, Office of Justice Programs, Bureau of Justice Statistics, *Sourcebook of Criminal Justice Statistics 1988* at 299, table 3.19 (1989). In 1988, an estimated 73 of every 100,000 females in the country were reported rape victims. Federal Bureau of Investigation, *Uniform Crime Reports for 1988* at 16 (1989).

11. Of course, where male employees allege that co-workers engage in conduct which creates a hostile environment, the appropriate victim's perspective would be that of a reasonable man.

ment.[12] *Andrews,* 895 F.2d at 1482 (sexual harassment must detrimentally affect a reasonable person of the same sex as the victim); *Yates,* 819 F.2d at 637 (adopting "reasonable woman" standard set out in *Rabidue,* 805 F.2d 611, 626 (Keith, J. dissenting)); Comment, *Sexual Harassment Claims of Abusive Work Environment Under Title VII,* 97 Harv.L.Rev. 1449, 1459 (1984); *cf. State v. Wanrow,* 88 Wash.2d 221, 239–241, 559 P.2d 548, 558–559 (1977) (en banc) (adopting reasonable woman standard for self defense).

We adopt the perspective of a reasonable woman primarily because we believe that a sex-blind reasonable person standard tends to be male-biased and tends to systematically ignore the experiences of women. The reasonable woman standard does not establish a higher level of protection for women than men. *Cf. Rosenfeld v. Southern Pacific Co.,* 444 F.2d 1219, 1225–1227 (9th Cir.1971) (invalidating under Title VII paternalistic state labor laws restricting employment opportunities for women). Instead, a gender-conscious examination of sexual harassment enables women to participate in the workplace on an equal footing with men. By acknowledging and not trivializing the effects of sexual harassment on reasonable women, courts can work towards ensuring that neither men nor women will have to "run a gauntlet of sexual abuse in return for the privilege of being allowed to work and make a living." *Henson v. Dundee,* 682 F.2d 897, 902 (11th Cir.1982).

We note that the reasonable victim standard we adopt today classifies conduct as unlawful sexual harassment even when harassers do not realize that their conduct creates a hostile working environment. Well-intentioned compliments by co-workers or supervisors can form the basis of a sexual harassment cause of action if a reasonable victim of the same sex as the plaintiff would consider the comments sufficiently severe or pervasive to alter a condition of employment and create an abusive working environment.[13] That is because Title VII is not a fault-based tort scheme. "Title VII is aimed at the consequences or effects of an employment practice and not at the . . . motivation" of co-workers or employers. *Rogers,* 454 F.2d at 239; *see also Griggs v. Duke Power Co.,* 401 U.S. 424, 432, 91 S.Ct. 849, 854, 28 L.Ed.2d 158 (1971) (the absence of discriminatory intent does not redeem an otherwise unlawful employment practice). To avoid liability under Title VII, employers may have to educate and sensitize their workforce to eliminate conduct which a reasonable victim would consider unlawful sexual harassment. *See* 29 C.F.R. § 1604.11(f) ("Prevention is the best tool for the elimination of sexual harassment").

---

12. We realize that the reasonable woman standard will not address conduct which some women find offensive. Conduct considered harmless by many today may be considered discriminatory in the future. *Rogers,* 454 F.2d at 238. Fortunately, the reasonableness inquiry which we adopt today is not static. As the views of reasonable women change, so too does the Title VII standard of acceptable behavior.

13. If sexual comments or sexual advances are in fact welcomed by the recipient, they, of course, do not constitute sexual harassment. Title VII's prohibition of sex discrimination in employment does not require a totally desexualized workplace.

The facts of this case illustrate the importance of considering the victim's perspective. Analyzing the facts from the alleged harasser's viewpoint, Gray could be portrayed as a modern-day Cyrano de Bergerac wishing no more than to woo Ellison with his words.[14] There is no evidence that Gray harbored ill will toward Ellison. He even offered in his "love letter" to leave her alone if she wished. Examined in this light, it is not difficult to see why the district court characterized Gray's conduct as isolated and trivial.

Ellison, however, did not consider the acts to be trivial. Gray's first note shocked and frightened her. After receiving the three-page letter, she became really upset and frightened again. She immediately requested that she or Gray be transferred. Her supervisor's prompt response suggests that she too did not consider the conduct trivial. When Ellison learned that Gray arranged to return to San Mateo, she immediately asked to transfer, and she immediately filed an official complaint.

[7] We cannot say as a matter of law that Ellison's reaction was idiosyncratic or hyper-sensitive. We believe that a reasonable woman could have had a similar reaction. After receiving the first bizarre note from Gray, a person she barely knew, Ellison asked a co-worker to tell Gray to leave her alone. Despite her request, Gray sent her a long, passionate, disturbing letter. He told her he had been "watching" and "experiencing" her; he made repeated references to sex; he said he would write again. Ellison had no way of knowing what Gray would do next. A reasonable woman could consider Gray's conduct, as alleged by Ellison, sufficiently severe and pervasive to alter a condition of employment and create an abusive working environment.

Sexual harassment is a major problem in the workplace.[15] Adopting the victim's perspective ensures that courts will not "sustain ingrained notions of reasonable behavior fashioned by the offenders." *Lipsett*, 864 F.2d at 898, *quoting*, *Rabidue*, 805 F.2d at 626 (Keith, J., dissenting). Congress did not enact Title VII to codify prevailing sexist prejudices. To the contrary, "Congress designed Title VII to prevent the perpetuation of stereotypes and a sense of degradation which serve to close or discourage employment opportunities for women." *Andrews*, 895 F.2d at 1483. We hope that over time both men and women will learn what conduct offends reasonable members of the other sex. When employers and employees

---

14. E. Rostand, *Cyrano de Bergerac* (B. Hooker trans. 1963).

15. Over 40 percent of female federal employees reported incidents of sexual harassment in 1987, roughly the same number as in 1980. United States Merit Systems Protection Board, *Sexual Harassment in the Federal Government: An Update* 11 (1988). Victims of sexual harassment "pay all the intangible emotional costs inflicted by anger, humiliation, frustration, withdrawal, dysfunction in family life," as well as medical expenses, litigation expenses, job search expenses, and the loss of valuable sick leave and annual leave. *Id.* at 42. Sexual harassment cost the federal government $267 million from May 1985 to May 1987 for losses in productivity, sick leave costs, and employee replacement costs. *Id.* at 39.

internalize the standard of workplace conduct we establish today, the current gap in perception between the sexes will be bridged.

IV

We next must determine what remedial actions by employers shield them from liability under Title VII for sexual harassment by co-workers. The Supreme Court in *Meritor* did not address employer liability for sexual harassment by co-workers. In that case, the Court discussed employer liability for a hostile environment created by a supervisor.

The Court's discussion was brief, and it declined to issue a definitive rule. 477 U.S. at 72, 106 S.Ct. at 2408. On one hand, it held that employers are not strictly liable for sexual harassment by supervisors. *Id.* On the other hand, it stated that employers can be liable for sexual harassment without actual notice of the alleged discriminatory conduct. *Id.* It agreed with the EEOC that courts should look to agency principles to determine liability. *Id.*

We applied *Meritor* in *E.E.O.C. v. Hacienda Hotel,* 881 F.2d 1504 (9th Cir.1989). We held that "employers are liable for failing to remedy or prevent a hostile or offensive work environment of which management-level employees knew, or in the exercise of reasonable care should have known." *Id.* at 1515–1516. Because management level employees at the hotel took no action to redress the sexual harassment of which they knew and other harassment of which they should have known, we held the employer liable. *Id.* at 1516. We have not addressed what remedial actions taken by employers can shield them from liability for sexual harassment by co-workers.

The EEOC guidelines recommend that an employer's remedy should be "immediate and appropriate." 29 C.F.R. § 1604.11(d).[16] Employers have a duty to "express[ ] strong disapproval" of sexual harassment, and to "develop[ ] appropriate sanctions." 29 C.F.R. § 1604.11(f). The EEOC explains that an employer's action is appropriate where it "fully remedie[s] the conduct without adversely affecting the terms or conditions of the charging party's employment in some manner (for example, by requiring the charging party to work . . . in a less desirable location)." EEOC Compliance Manual (CCH) § 615.4(a)(9)(iii), ¶ 3103, at 3213 (1988).

The Fourth Circuit has required that a remedy be "reasonably calculated to end the harassment." *Katz v. Dole,* 709 F.2d 251, 256 (4th Cir.1983). It has held that an employer properly remedied sexual harassment by fully investigating the allegations, issuing written warnings to refrain from discriminatory conduct, and warn-

---

16. That regulation states: "With respect to conduct between fellow employees, an employer is responsible for acts of sexual harassment in the workplace where the employer (or its agents or supervisory employees) knows or should have known of the conduct, unless it can show that it took immediate and appropriate corrective action."

ing the offender that a subsequent infraction will result in suspension. *Swentek v. USAIR, Inc.,* 830 F.2d 552 (4th Cir.1987).

Similarly, in *Barrett v. Omaha National Bank,* 726 F.2d 424, 427 (8th Cir.1984), the Eighth Circuit held that an employer properly remedied a hostile working environment by fully investigating, reprimanding a harasser for grossly inappropriate conduct, placing the offender on probation for ninety days, and warning the offender that any further misconduct would result in discharge. The court concluded that Title VII does not require employers to fire all harassers.

[8] We too believe that remedies should be "reasonably calculated to end the harassment." *Katz,* 709 F.2d at 256. An employer's remedy should persuade individual harassers to discontinue unlawful conduct. We do not think that all harassment warrants dismissal, *Barrett,* 726 F.2d at 427; rather, remedies should be "assessed proportionately to the seriousness of the offense." *Dornhecker v. Malibu Grand Prix Corp.,* 828 F.2d 307, 309 (5th Cir.1987). Employers should impose sufficient penalties to assure a workplace free from sexual harassment. In essence, then, we think that the reasonableness of an employer's remedy will depend on its ability to stop harassment by the person who engaged in harassment.[17] In evaluating the adequacy of the remedy, the court may also take into account the remedy's ability to persuade potential harassers to refrain from unlawful conduct. Indeed, meting out punishments that do not take into account the need to maintain a harassment-free working environment may subject the employer to suit by the EEOC.

[9] Here, Ellison's employer argues that it complied with its statutory obligation to provide a workplace free from sexual harassment. It promptly investigated Ellison's allegation. When Ellison returned to San Mateo from her training in St. Louis, Gray was no longer working in San Mateo. When Gray returned to San Mateo, the government granted Ellison's request to transfer temporarily to San Francisco.

We decline to accept the government's argument that its decision to return Gray to San Mateo did not create a hostile environment for Ellison because the government granted Ellison's request for a temporary transfer to San Francisco. Ellison preferred to work in San Mateo over San Francisco. We strongly believe that the victim of sexual harassment should not be punished for the conduct of the harasser. We wholeheartedly agree with the EEOC that a victim of sexual harassment should not have to work in a less desirable location as a result of an

---

17. We do not think that the appropriate inquiry is what a reasonable employer would do to remedy the sexual harassment. *Contra Brooms v. Regal Tube Co.,* 881 F.2d 412, 421 (7th Cir.1989). Although employers are statutorily obligated to provide a workplace free from sexual harassment, they may be reluctant, for business reasons, to punish high ranking and highly productive employees for sexual harassment. In addition, asking what a reasonable employer would do runs the risk of reinforcing any prevailing level of discrimination by employers and fails to focus directly on the best way to eliminate sexual harassment from the workplace.

employer's remedy for sexual harassment. EEOC Compliance Manual (CCH) § 615.4(a)(9)(iii), ¶ 3103, at 3213 (1988).

Ellison maintains that the government's remedy was insufficient because it did not discipline Gray and because it allowed Gray to return to San Mateo after only a six-month separation. Even though the hostile environment had been eliminated when Gray began working in San Francisco, we cannot say that the government's response was reasonable under Title VII. The record on appeal suggests that Ellison's employer did not express strong disapproval of Gray's conduct, did not reprimand Gray, did not put him on probation, and did not inform him that repeated harassment would result in suspension or termination. *Cf. Swentek*, 830 F.2d 552; *Barrett*, 726 F.2d 424. Apparently, Gray's employer only told him to stop harassing Ellison.[18] Title VII requires more than a mere request to refrain from discriminatory conduct. *DeGrace v. Rumsfeld*, 614 F.2d 796, 805 n. 5 (1st Cir.1980). Employers send the wrong message to potential harassers when they do not discipline employees for sexual harassment. If Ellison can prove on remand that Gray knew or should have known that his conduct was unlawful and that the government failed to take even the mildest form of disciplinary action, the district court should hold that the government's initial remedy was insufficient under Title VII. At this point, genuine issues of material fact remain concerning whether the government properly disciplined Gray.

Ellison further maintains that her employer's decision to allow Gray to transfer back to the San Mateo office after a six-month cooling-off period rendered the government's remedy insufficient. She argues that Gray's *mere presence* would create a hostile working environment.

[10] We believe that in some cases the mere presence of an employee who has engaged in particularly severe or pervasive harassment can create a hostile working environment. *See Paroline v. Unisys Corp.*, 879 F.2d 100, 106–07 (4th Cir.1989). To avoid liability under Title VII for failing to remedy a hostile environment, employers may even have to remove employees from the workplace if their mere presence would render the working environment hostile.[19] Once again, we examine whether

---

18. Neither the counseling session with Miller nor Gray's transfer to San Francisco was a disciplinary act by the IRS.

19. If harassers are not removed from the workplace when their mere presence creates a hostile environment, employers have not fully remedied the harassment. When employers cannot schedule harassers to work at another location or during different hours, employers may have to dismiss employees whose mere presence creates a hostile environment. We acknowledge that in rare instances dismissal may be necessary when harassers did not realize that their conduct was unlawful. However, we think that only in very, very few cases will harassers be unaware that their conduct is unlawful when that conduct is so serious that a reasonable victim would thereafter consider the harasser's mere presence sexual harassment. In those few instances, we think it only proper to conclude that the harasser should have known that his or her conduct was unlawful.

In order to avoid the loss of well-intentioned productive employees, employers must educate and sensitize their workforce.

the mere presence of a harasser would create a hostile environment from the perspective of a reasonable woman.

The district court did not reach the issue of the reasonableness of the government's remedy. Given the scant record on appeal, we cannot determine whether a reasonable woman could conclude that Gray's mere presence at San Mateo six months after the alleged harassment would create an abusive environment. Although we are aware of the severity of Gray's conduct (which we do not consider to be as serious as some other forms of harassment), we do not know how often Ellison and Gray would have to interact at San Mateo.

Moreover, it is not clear to us that the six-month cooling-off period was reasonably calculated to end the harassment or assessed proportionately to the seriousness of Gray's conduct. There is evidence in the record which suggests that the government intended to transfer Gray to San Francisco permanently and only allowed Gray to return to San Mateo because he promised to drop some union grievances. We do know that the IRS did not request Ellison's input or even inform her of the proceedings before agreeing to let Gray return to San Mateo. This failure to even attempt to determine what impact Gray's return would have on Ellison shows an insufficient regard for the victim's interest in avoiding a hostile working environment. On remand, the district court should fully explore the facts concerning the government's decision to return Gray to San Mateo.[20]

V

We reverse the district court's decision that Ellison did not allege a prima facie case of sexual harassment due to a hostile working environment, and we remand for further proceedings consistent with this opinion. Although we have considered the evidence in the light most favorable to Ellison because the district court granted the government's motion for summary judgment, we, of course, reserve for the district court the resolution of all factual issues.

Reversed and remanded.

Stephens, District Judge, dissenting:

This case comes to us on appeal in the wake of the granting of a summary judgment motion. There was no trial, therefore no opportunities for cross exami-

---

20. We note that if the district court decides that the government's actions were not reasonably calculated to end the harassment or assessed proportionately to the seriousness of the conduct, Ellison's relief will be primarily injunctive. Title VII does not provide for compensatory or punitive damages. See *Williams v. United States General Services Administration*, 905 F.2d 308, 311 (9th Cir.1990).

In the event that the district court decides to award Ellison equitable relief, the court should not fail to consider any relevant commitments made by the government in Gray's settlement agreement.

nation of the witnesses. In addition, there are factual gaps in the record that can only lead by speculation. Consequently, I believe that it is an inappropriate case with which to establish a new legal precedent which will be binding in all subsequent cases of like nature in the Ninth Circuit. I refer to the majority's use of the term "reasonable woman," a term I find ambiguous and therefore inadequate.

Nowhere in section 2000e of Title VII, the section under which the plaintiff in this case brought suit, is there any indication that Congress intended to provide for any other than equal treatment in the area of civil rights. The legislation is designed to achieve a balanced and generally gender neutral and harmonious workplace which would improve production and the quality of the employees' lives. In fact, the Supreme Court has shown a preference against systems that are not gender or race neutral, such as hiring quotas. *See City of Richmond v. J.A. Croson Co.,* 488 U.S. 469, 109 S.Ct. 706, 102 L.Ed.2d 854 (1989). While women may be the most frequent targets of this type of conduct that is at issue in this case, they are not the only targets. I believe that it is incumbent upon the court in this case to use terminology that will meet the needs of all who seek recourse under this section of Title VII. Possible alternatives that are more in line with a gender neutral approach include "victim," "target," or "person."

The term "reasonable man" as it is used in the law of torts, traditionally refers to the average adult person, regardless of gender, and the conduct that can reasonably be expected of him or her. For the purposes of the legal issues that are being addressed, such a term assumes that it is applicable to all persons. Section 2000e of Title VII presupposes the use of a legal term that can apply to all persons and the impossibility of a more individually tailored standard. It is clear that the authors of the majority opinion intend a difference between the "reasonable woman" and the "reasonable man" in Title VII cases on the assumption that men do not have the same sensibilities as women. This is not necessarily true. A man's response to circumstances faced by women and their effect upon women can be and in given circumstances may be expected to be understood by men.

It takes no stretch of the imagination to envision two complaints emanating from the same workplace regarding the same conditions, one brought by a woman and the other by a man. Application of the "new standard" presents a puzzlement which is born of the assumption that men's eyes do not see what a woman sees through her eyes. I find it surprising that the majority finds no need for evidence on any of these subjects. I am not sure whether the majority also concludes that the woman and the man in question are also reasonable without evidence on this subject. I am irresistibly drawn to the view that the conditions of the workplace itself should be examined as affected, among other things, by the conduct of the people working there as to whether the workplace as existing is conducive to fulfilling the goals of Title VII. In any event, these are unresolved factual issues which preclude summary judgment.

The focus on the victim of the sexually discriminatory conduct has its parallel in rape trials in the focus put by the defense on the victim's conduct rather than on the unlawful conduct of the person accused. Modern feminists have pointed out that concentration by the defense upon evidence concerning the background, appearance and conduct of women claiming to have been raped must be carefully controlled by the court to avoid effectively shifting the burden of proof to the victim. It is the accused, not the victim who is on trial, and it is therefore the conduct of the accused, not that of the victim, that should be subjected to scrutiny.[1] Many state legislatures have responded to this viewpoint, and rules governing the presentation of evidence in rape cases have evolved accordingly.[2] *See generally*, Galvin, Shielding Rape Victims in the State and Federal Courts: a Proposal for the Second Decade, 70 Minn.L.Rev. 763 (April 1986).

It is my opinion that the case should be reversed with instructions to proceed to trial. This would certainly lead to filling in the factual gaps left by the scanty record, such as what happened at the time of or after the visit of Ellison to Gray's house to cause her to be subsequently fearful of his presence. The circumstances existing in the work place where only men are employed are different than they are where there are both male and female employees. The existence of the differences is readily recognizable and the conduct of employees can be changed appropriately. This is what Title VII requires. Whether a man or a woman has sensibilities peculiar to the person and what they are is not necessarily known. Until they become known by manifesting themselves in an obvious way, they do not become part of the circumstances of the work place. Consequently, the governing element in the equation is the workplace itself, not concepts or viewpoints of individual employees. This does not conflict with existing legal concepts.

The creation of the proposed "new standard" which applies only to women will not necessarily come to the aid of all potential victims of the type of misconduct that is at issue in this case. I believe that a gender neutral standard would greatly contribute to the clarity of this and future cases in the same area.

Summary judgment is not appropriate in this case.

---

[1] *Cf. People v. Rioz*, 161 Cal.App.3d 905, 909–910, 207 Cal.Rptr. 903, 916 (1984) (evidence of whether the victim engaged in sexual activity with numerous men, even for pecuniary gain, is controlled by the procedural safeguards in evidentiary law).

[2] *See* Fed.R.Civ.Pro. 412; Vhay, The Harms of Asking: Towards a Comprehensive Treatment of Sexual Harassment, 55 U.Chi.L.Rev. 328, 345, n. 78 (Winter 1988); Fechner, Toward an Expanded Conception of Law Reform: Sexual Harassment Law and the Reconstruction of Facts, 23 U.Mich.J.L.Ref. 475, 495 (Spring 1990).

## HARRIS V. FORKLIFT SYSTEMS

# SUPREME COURT OF THE UNITED STATES

No. 92–1168

TERESA HARRIS, PETITIONER v. FORKLIFT SYSTEMS, INC.

**on writ of certiorari to the United States Court of Appeals for the Sixth Circuit**
**November 9, 1993**

Justice O'Connor delivered the opinion of the Court.

In this case we consider the definition of a discriminatorily "abusive work environment" (also known as a "hostile work environment") under Title VII of the Civil Rights Act of 1964, 78 Stat. 253, as amended, 42 U.S.C. 2000e *et seq.* (1988 ed., Supp. III).

I

Teresa Harris worked as a manager at Forklift Systems, Inc., an equipment rental company, from April 1985 until October 1987. Charles Hardy was Forklift's president.

The Magistrate found that, throughout Harris' time at Forklift, Hardy often insulted her because of her gender and often made her the target of unwanted sexual innuendos. Hardy told Harris on several occasions, in the presence of other employees, "You're a woman, what do you know" and "We need a man as the rental manager"; at least once, he told her she was "a dumb ass woman." App. to Pet. for Cert. A–13. Again in front of others, he suggested that the two of them "go to the Holiday Inn to negotiate [Harris'] raise." *Id.,* at A–14. Hardy occasionally asked Harris and other female employees to get coins from his front pants pocket. *Ibid.* He threw objects on the ground in front of Harris and other women, and asked them to pick the objects up. *Id.,* at A–14 to A–15. He made sexual innuendos about Harris' and other women's clothing. *Id.,* at A–15.

In mid-August 1987, Harris complained to Hardy about his conduct. Hardy said he was surprised that Harris was offended, claimed he was only joking, and apologized. *Id.,* at A–16. He also promised he would stop, and based on this assurance Harris stayed on the job. *Ibid.* But in early September, Hardy began anew: While Harris was arranging a deal with one of Forklift's customers, he asked her, again in front of other employees, "What did you do, promise the guy . . . some [sex] Saturday night?" *Id.,* at A–17. On October 1, Harris collected her paycheck and quit.

Harris then sued Forklift, claiming that Hardy's conduct had created an abusive work environment for her because of her gender. The United States District Court for the Middle District of Tennessee, adopting the report and recommendation of the Magistrate, found this to be "a close case," *id.*, at A–31, but held that Hardy's conduct did not create an abusive environment. The court found that some of Hardy's comments "offended [Harris], and would offend the reasonable woman," *id.*, at A–33, but that they were not "so severe as to be expected to seriously affect [Harris'] psychological well-being. A reasonable woman manager under like circumstances would have been offended by Hardy, but his conduct would not have risen to the level of interfering with that person's work performance.

"Neither do I believe that [Harris] was subjectively so offended that she suffered injury. . . . Although Hardy may at times have genuinely offended [Harris], I do not believe that he created a working environment so poisoned as to be intimidating or abusive to [Harris]." *Id.*, at A–34 to A–35.

In focusing on the employee's psychological well-being, the District Court was following Circuit precedent. See *Rabidue v. Osceola Refining Co.*, 805 F.2d 611, 620 (CA6 1986), cert. denied, 481 U.S. 1041, 107 S.Ct.1983, 95 L.Ed.2d 823 (1987). The United States Court of Appeals for the Sixth Circuit affirmed in a brief unpublished decision, 976 F.2d 733 (CA6 1992).

We granted certiorari, 507 U.S.——, 113 S.Ct. 1382, 122 L.Ed.2d 758 (1993), to resolve a conflict among the Circuits on whether conduct, to be actionable as "abusive work environment" harassment (no *quid pro quo* harassment issue is present here), must "seriously affect [an employee's] psychological well-being" or lead the plaintiff to "suffe[r] injury." Compare *Rabidue* (requiring serious effect on psychological well-being); *Vance v. Southern Bell Telephone & Telegraph Co.*, 863 F.2d 1503, 1510 (CA11 1989) (same); and *Downes v FAA*, 775 F.2d 288, 292 (CA Fed.1985) (same), with *Ellison v. Brady*, 924 F.2d 872, 877–878 (CA9 1991) (rejecting such a requirement).

II

[1, 2] Title VII of the Civil Rights Act of 1964 makes it "an unlawful employment practice for an employer . . . to discriminate against any individual with respect to his compensation, terms, conditions, or privileges of employment, because of such individual's race, color, religion, sex, or national origin." 42 U.S.C. § 2000e–2(a)(1). As we made clear in *Meritor Savings Bank v. Vinson*, 477 U.S. 57, 106 S.Ct. 2399, 91 L.Ed.2d 49 (1986), this language "is not limited to 'economic' or 'tangible' discrimination. The phrase 'terms, conditions, or privileges of employment' evinces a congressional intent 'to strike at the entire spectrum of disparate treatment of men and women' in employment," which includes requiring people to work in a discriminatorily hostile or abusive environment. *Id.*, at 64, 104 S.Ct., at 2404, quoting *Los Angeles Dept. of Water and Power v. Manhart*, 435 U.S. 702, 707, n. 13, 98 S.Ct. 1370, 1374, 55 L.Ed.2d 657 (1978) (some internal quota-

tion marks omitted). When the workplace is permeated with "discriminatory intimidation, ridicule, and insult," 477 U.S., at 65, 106 S.Ct., at 2405, that is "sufficiently severe or pervasive to alter the conditions of the victim's employment and create an abusive working environment," *id.*, at 67, 106 S.Ct., at 2403 (internal brackets and quotation marks omitted), Title VII is violated.

[3] This standard, which we reaffirm today, takes a middle path between making actionable any conduct that is merely offensive and requiring the conduct to cause a tangible psychological injury. As we pointed out in *Meritor*, "mere utterance of an . . . epithet which engenders offensive feelings in a employee," *ibid.* (internal quotation marks omitted) does not sufficiently affect the conditions of employment to implicate Title VII. Conduct that is not severe or pervasive enough to create an objectively hostile or abusive work environment—an environment that a reasonable person would find hostile or abusive—is beyond Title VII's purview. Likewise, if the victim does not subjectively perceive the environment to be abusive, the conduct has not actually altered the conditions of the victim's employment, and there is no Title VII violation.

[4, 5] But Title VII comes into play before the harassing conduct leads to a nervous breakdown. A discriminatorily abusive work environment, even one that does not seriously affect employees' psychological well-being, can and often will detract from employees' job performance, discourage employees from remaining on the job, or keep them from advancing in their careers. Moreover, even without regard to these tangible effects, the very fact that the discriminatory conduct was so severe or pervasive that it created a work environment abusive to employees because of their race, gender, religion, or national origin offends Title VII's broad rule of workplace equality. The appalling conduct alleged in *Meritor*, and the reference in that case to environments " 'so heavily polluted with discrimination as to destroy completely the emotional and psychological stability of minority group workers,' " *supra*, at 66, 106 S.Ct., at 2405, quoting *Rogers v. EEOC*, 454 F.2d 234, 238 (CA5 1971), cert. denied, 406 U.S. 957, 92 S.Ct. 2058, 32 L.Ed.2d 343 (1972), merely present some especially egregious examples of harassment. They do not mark the boundary of what is actionable.

[6] We therefore believe the District Court erred in relying on whether the conduct "seriously affect[ed] plaintiff's psychological well-being" or led her to "suffe[r] injury." Such an inquiry may needlessly focus the factfinder's attention on concrete psychological harm, an element Title VII does not require. Certainly Title VII bars conduct that would seriously affect a reasonable person's psychological well-being, but the statute is not limited to such conduct. So long as the environment would reasonably be perceived, and is perceived, as hostile or abusive, *Meritor, supra*, 477 U.S., at 67, 106 S.Ct., at 2045, there is no need for it also to be psychologically injurious.

[7] This is not, and by its nature cannot be, a mathematically precise test. We need not answer today all the potential questions it raises, nor specifically address

the EEOC's new regulations on this subject, see 58 Fed. Reg. 51266 (1993) (proposed 29 CFR §§ 1609.1, 1609.2); see also 29 CFR § 1604.11 (1993). But we can say that whether an environment is "hostile" or "abusive" can be determined only by looking at all the circumstances. These may include the frequency of the discriminatory conduct; its severity; whether it is physically threatening or humiliating, or a mere offensive utterance; and whether it unreasonably interferes with an employee's work performance. The effect on the employee's psychological well-being is, of course, relevant to determining whether the plaintiff actually found the environment abusive. But while psychological harm, like any other relevant factor, may be taken into account, no single factor is required.

III

[8] Forklift, while conceding that a requirement that the conduct seriously affect psychological well-being is unfounded, argues that the District Court nonetheless correctly applied the *Meritor* standard. We disagree. Though the District Court did conclude that the work environment was not "intimidating or abusive to [Harris]," App. to Pet. for Cert. A–35, it did so only after finding that the conduct was not "so severe as to be expected to seriously affect plaintiff's psychological well-being," *id.*, at A–34, and that Harris was not "subjectively so offended that she suffered injury," *ibid.* The District Court's application of these incorrect standards may well have influenced its ultimate conclusion, especially given that the court found this to be a "close case," *id.*, at A–31.

We therefore reverse the judgment of the Court of Appeals, and remand the case for further proceedings consistent with this opinion.

*So ordered.*

# SUPREME COURT OF THE UNITED STATES

---

No. 92-1168

---

TERESA HARRIS, PETITIONER v. FORKLIFT SYSTEMS, INC.

**on writ of certiorari to the United States Court of Appeals for the Sixth Circuit**
**November 9, 1993**

Justice Ginsburg, concurring.

Today the Court reaffirms the holding of *Meritor Savings Bank v. Vinson*, 477 U.S. 57, 66, 106 S.Ct. 2399, 2405, 91 L.Ed.2d 49 (1986): "[A] plaintiff may establish a violation of Title VII by proving that discrimination based on sex has created a hostile or abusive work environment." The critical issue, Title VII's text indicates, is whether members of one sex are exposed to disadvantageous terms or conditions of employment to which members of the other sex are not exposed. See 42 U.S.C. § 2000e–2(a)(1) (declaring that it is unlawful to discriminate with respect to, *inter alia*, "terms" or "conditions" of employment). As the Equal Employment Opportunity Commission emphasized, see Brief for United States and Equal Employment Opportunity Commission as *Amici Curiae* 9–14, the adjudicator's inquiry should center, dominantly, on whether the discriminatory conduct has unreasonably interfered with the plaintiff's work performance. To show such interference, "the plaintiff need not prove that his or her tangible productivity has declined as a result of the harassment." *Davis v. Monsanto Chemical Co.,* 858 F.2d 345, 349 (CA6 1988). It suffices to prove that a reasonable person subjected to the discriminatory conduct would find, as the plaintiff did, that the harassment so altered working conditions as to "ma[k]e it more difficult to do the job." See *ibid. Davis* concerned race-based discrimination, but that difference does not alter the analysis; except in the rare case in which a bona fide occupational qualification is shown, see *Automobile Workers v. Johnson Controls, Inc.,* 499 U.S. 187, 200–207 (1991) (construing 42 U.S.C. 2000e–2(e)(1)), Title VII declares discriminatory practices based on race, gender, religion, or national origin equally unlawful.

The Court's opinion, which I join, seems to me in harmony with the view expressed in this concurring statement.

## SUPREME COURT OF THE UNITED STATES

No. 92-1168

TERESA HARRIS, PETITIONER V. FORKLIFT SYSTEMS, INC.

**on writ of certiorari to the United States Court of Appeals for the Sixth Circuit**
**November 9, 1993**

Justice Scalia, concurring.

*Meritor Savings Bank v. Vinson,* 477 U.S. 57, 106 S.Ct. 2399, 91 L.Ed.2d 49 (1986), held that Title VII prohibits sexual harassment that takes the form of a hostile work environment. The Court states that sexual harassment is actionable if it is "sufficiently severe or pervasive 'to alter the conditions of [the victim's] employment and create an abusive work environment.'" *Id.,* at 67, 106 S.Ct., at 2045 (quoting *Henson v. Dundee,* 682 F.2d 897, 904 (CA11 1982)). Today's opinion elaborates that the challenged conduct must be severe or pervasive enough "to create an objectively hostile or abusive work environment—an environment that a reasonable person would find hostile or abusive." *Ante,* at 370.

"Abusive" (or "hostile," which in this context I take to mean the same thing) does not seem to me a very clear standard—and I do not think clarity is at all increased by adding the adverb "objectively" or by appealing to a "reasonable person's" notion of what the vague word means. Today's opinion does list a number of factors that contribute to abusiveness, see *ante*, at 371, but since it neither says how much of each is necessary (an impossible task) nor identifies any single factor as determinative, it thereby adds little certitude. As a practical matter, today's holding lets virtually unguided juries decide whether sex-related conduct engaged in (or permitted by) an employer is egregious enough to warrant an award of damages. One might say that what constitutes "negligence" (a traditional jury question) is not much more clear and certain than what constitutes "abusiveness." Perhaps so. But the class of plaintiffs seeking to recover for negligence is limited to those who have suffered harm, whereas under this statute "abusiveness" is to be the test of whether legal harm has been suffered, opening more expansive vistas of litigation.

Be that as it may, I know of no alternative to the course the Court today has taken. One of the factors mentioned in the Court's nonexhaustive list—whether the conduct unreasonably interferes with an employee's work performance—would, if it were made an absolute test, provide greater guidance to juries and employers. But I see no basis for such a limitation in the language of the statute. Accepting *Meritor*'s interpretation of the term "conditions of employment" as the law, the test is not whether work has been impaired, but whether working conditions have been discriminatorily altered. I know of no test more faithful to the inherently vague statutory language than the one the Court today adopts. For these reasons, I join the opinion of the Court.

# APPENDIX E
# BIBLIOGRAPHY

American Association of University Women. *Hostile Hallways: The AAUW Survey on Sexual Harassment in America's Schools*. Washington, DC: AAUW Educational Foundation, 1993.

Brown, Lyn Mikel, and Carol Gilligan. *Meeting at the Crossroads: Women's Psychology and Girls' Development*. New York: Ballantine, 1993.

Brownmiller, Susan, and Dolores Alexander. "From Carmita Wood to Anita Hill." *Ms.* magazine, vol. 2, no. 4 (1992), pp. 70–71.

*Civil Rights Act of 1964, Title VII.* 42 United States Code § 2000e.

Cooper-White, Pamela. *The Cry of Tamar: Violence Against Women and the Church's Response*. Minneapolis: Fortress Press, 1995.

*Corne v. Bausch & Lomb.* 390 F.Supp. 161 (D. Ariz. 1975).

Culbertson, Amy L., and Paul Rosenfeld. "Assessment of Sexual Harassment in the Active-duty Navy." *Military Psychology* (Special Issue: Women in the Navy), vol. 6 (1994), pp. 69–93.

Dewar, Helen. "Panel Details Packwood Allegations." *Washington Post*, May 18, 1995.

Ellis, Bruce J., and Donald Symons. "Sex Differences in Sexual Fantasy: An Evolutionary Psychological Approach." *Journal of Sex Research*, vol. 27 (1990), pp. 527–555.

*Ellison v. Brady*. 924 F.2d 872 (9th Cir. 1991).

Equal Employment Opportunity Commission (EEOC). "Guidelines on Discrimination Because of Sex." 29 C.F.R.1604, 1980.

Farley, Lin. *Sexual Shakedown*. New York: Warner Books, 1978.

Fitzgerald, Louise F., and Alayne J. Ormerod. "Perceptions of Sexual Harassment: The Influence of Gender and Academic Context." *Psychology of Women Quarterly*, vol. 15, no. 2 (June 1991).

Freeman, Jo. "How 'Sex' Got Into Title VII: Persistent Opportunism as a Maker of Public Policy." *Law and Inequality: A Journal of Theory and Practice*, vol. 9 (1991), pp. 163–84.

Gilligan, Carol. *In a Different Voice: Psychological Theory and Women's Development*. Cambridge: Harvard University Press, 1982.

Gilligan, Carol, Annie G. Rogers, and Deborah L. Tolman, eds. *Women, Girls and Psychotherapy: Reframing Resistance*. New York: Haworth Press, 1991.

Gruber, James E. "A Typology of Personal and Environmental Sexual Harassment: Research and Policy Implications for the 1990s." *Sex Roles: A Journal of Research*, vol. 26, no. 11–12 (June 1992).

Gutek, Barbara A. "Responses to Sexual Harassment." In Stuart Oskamp and Mark Costanzo, eds., *Gender Issues in Contemporary Society*. Newbury Park, CA: Sage Publications, 1993.

Gutek, Barbara A., and Aaron G. Cohen. "Sex Ratios, Sex Role Spillover, and Sex at Work: A Comparison of Men's and Women's Experiences." *Human Relations*, vol. 40 (1987), pp. 97–115.

Gutek, Barbara A., and Mary P. Koss. "Changed Women and Changed Organizations: Consequences of and Coping with Sexual Harassment." *Journal of Vocational Behavior* (Special Issue: Sexual Harassment in the Workplace), vol. 42 (1993), pp. 29–39.

Harding, M. Esther. *The Way of All Women*. New York: Putnam, 1971.

*Harris v. Forklift Systems*. 114 S.Ct.367 (1993).

Herman, Judith Lewis. *Trauma and Recovery*. New York: Basic Books, 1992.

Hippensteele, Susan. "Advocacy and Student Victims of Sexual Harassment." In B. Sandler and R. Shoop, eds., *Sexual Harassment on Campus: A Guide for Administrators, Faculty and Students*. Boston: Allyn and Bacon, 1996.

Holden, Benjamin A. "Hilton Hotels Loses $5 Million Verdict in Tailhook Case." *Wall Street Journal*, Nov. 1, 1994.

Hughes, Jean O'Gorman, and Bernice R. Sandler. *"Friends" Raping Friends: Could It Happen to You?* Washington, DC: Project on the Status and Education of Women, Association of American Colleges, 1987.

Jung, C. G. *Memories, Dreams, Reflections*. New York: Vintage Books, 1989.

Jung, C. G. *Two Essays on Analytical Psychology*. 2d ed. Princeton: Princeton University Press, 1966.

Kemp, Susan G., Richard J. Curiale, and Stephen J. Hirschfeld. *Stopping Sexual Harassment: An Employer's Guide*. Sacramento: California Chamber of Commerce, 1993.

Koss, Mary P., et al. *No Safe Haven: Male Violence Against Women at Home, at Work, and in the Community*. Washington, DC: American Psychological Association, 1994.

Lach, Denise, and Patricia A. Gwartney-Gibbs. "Sociological Perspectives on Sexual Harassment and Workplace Dispute Resolution." *Journal of Vocational Behavior* (Special Issue: Sexual Harassment in the Workplace), vol. 42 (1993), pp. 102–15.

Lewin, Tamar. "Chevron Agrees to Pay $2.2 Million in Settlement of Sexual Harassment Case." *New York Times*, Feb. 22, 1995.

Lindgren, J. Ralph, and Nadine Taub. *The Law of Sex Discrimination*. 2d ed. Minneapolis/St. Paul: West Publishing Co., 1993.

MacKinnon, Catharine A. *Sexual Harassment of Working Women: A Case of Sex Discrimination*. New Haven: Yale University Press, 1979.

*Meritor v. Vinson.* 477 U.S. 57 (1986).

Monson, Melissa. "Defining the Situation: Sexual Harassment or Everyday Rudeness?" Paper presented at the Conference of the Sociologists Against Sexual Harassment, 1994.

Nemy, Enid. "Women Begin to Speak Out Against Sexual Harassment at Work." *New York Times,* Aug. 19, 1975.

Orenstein, Peggy. *School Girls: Young Women, Self-Esteem, and the Confidence Gap.* New York: Doubleday, 1994.

Petrocelli, William, and Barbara Kate Repa. *Sexual Harassment on the Job: What It Is and How to Stop It.* 2d ed. Berkeley: Nolo Press, 1994.

Pipher, Mary. *Reviving Ophelia: Saving the Selves of Adolescent Girls.* New York: Ballantine, 1994.

Prozan, Charlotte Krause. *Feminist Psychoanalytic Psychotherapy.* Northvale, NJ: Jason Aronson, 1992.

Pryor, John B., Christine M. LaVite, and Lynnette M. Stoller. "A Social Psychological Analysis of Sexual Harassment: The Person/Situation Interaction." *Journal of Vocational Behavior* (Special Issue: Sexual Harassment in the Workplace), vol. 42, (1993), pp. 68–83.

Riger, Stephanie. "Gender Dilemmas in Sexual Harassment: Policies and Procedures." In Sherri Marie Matteo, ed., *American Women in the Nineties: Today's Critical Issues.* Boston: Northeastern University Press, 1993, pp. 213–34.

Rutter, Peter. *Sex in the Forbidden Zone: When Men in Power—Therapists, Doctors, Clergy, Teachers, and Others—Betray Women's Trust.* New York: Fawcett Crest, 1991.

Rutter, Virginia Beane. *Woman Changing Woman: Feminine Psychology Re-conceived Through Myth and Experience.* San Francisco: HarperSanFrancisco, 1993.

Samuels, Andrew. *Jung and the Post-Jungians.* New York: Routledge, 1985.

Shoop, Julie Gannon. "Beyond Horseplay: Students Sue Schools Over Sexual Harassment." *Trial,* vol. 30 (1994).

Stambaugh, Phoebe Morgan. "The Promise of Law: Understanding the Sexual Harassment Complaint Careers of Women." Arizona State University: Unpublished dissertation, 1995.

Stein, Nan D., and Lisa Sjostrom. *Flirting or Hurting: A Teacher's Guide on Student-to-Student Sexual Harassment in Schools.* Washington, DC: National Education Association, 1994.

Tannen, Deborah. *Talking from 9 to 5.* New York: William Morrow, 1994.

Tannen, Deborah. *You Just Don't Understand: Women and Men in Conversation.* New York: Ballantine, 1991.

U.S. Merit Systems Protection Board. "Employee Responses to Harassment." In *Sexual Harassment of Federal Workers: An Update.* Washington, DC: U.S. Government Printing Office, 1988.

*Williams v. Saxbe.* 413 F.Supp. 654 (D.D.C. 1976).

Zimmerman, Jean. *Tailspin: Women at War in the Wake of Tailhook.* New York: Doubleday, 1995.

# CHAPTER NOTES

Chapter I: Sexual Harassment: Psychology, Law, and the Reasonable Woman and Reasonable Man

P. 5 "about 90 percent of harassment episodes . . .": The largest government study to date found that only 5 percent of harassed workers made official complaints. See U.S. Merit Systems Protection Board, "Employee Responses to Harassment," in *Sexual Harassment of Federal Workers: An Update* (Washington, DC: U.S. Government Printing Office, 1988), chap. 3. The full text of this document is available on the Internet. See this book's World Wide Web site (**http: //www.bdd.com/rutter**) for the link. A study of U.S. Navy personnel found that 5 percent of female officers and 12 percent of enlisted women who felt they had been harassed filed a grievance. See Amy L. Culbertson and Paul Rosenfeld, "Assessment of Sexual Harassment in the Active-duty Navy," *Military Psychology* (Special Issue: Women in the Navy), vol. 6 (1994), pp. 69–93. A good overview of this subject with additional references can be found in: Barbara A. Gutek and Mary P. Koss, "Changed Women and Changed Organizations: Consequences of and Coping with Sexual Harassment," *Journal of Vocational Behavior* (Special Issue: Sexual Harassment in the Workplace), vol. 42 (1993), pp. 29–39.

P. 5 "a negative emotional and job-related impact": For a good overview of the research, see Denise Lach and Patricia A. Gwartney-Gibbs, "Sociological Perspectives on Sexual Harassment and Workplace Dispute Resolution," *Journal of Vocational Behavior* (Special Issue: Sexual Harassment in the Workplace), vol. 42 (1993), pp. 102–15. In her recent research, Phoebe Morgan Stambaugh followed thirty-two women through the complaint process and documented the many negative consequences. See Phoebe Morgan Stambaugh, "The Promise of Law: Understanding the Sexual Harassment Complaint Careers of Women" (Arizona State University: Unpublished dissertation, 1995).

P. 6 "We adopt the perspective of the reasonable woman . . .": From the Court's opinion in *Ellison v. Brady*, U.S. Court of Appeals, Ninth Circuit. The full text can be found in Appendix D of this book. This passage appears on page 215. The standard legal citation is 924 F.2d 872 (9th Cir.1991), p. 879.

P. 6 "would be that of a reasonable man": *Ellison v. Brady*, p. 214n.

## Chapter 2: Sex, Power, and Boundaries: Mapping the Territory

P. 9 "Farley describes how she and her colleagues . . .": Lin Farley, *Sexual Shakedown* (New York: Warner Books, 1978), pp. 11–12. Farley explains adopting this term for her 1974 course: "Each of us had already been fired from a job at least once because we had been made too uncomfortable by the behavior of men. . . . The male behavior eventually required a name, and *sexual harassment* seemed to come as close to symbolizing the problem as the language would permit." Also: "Farley and two Cornell colleagues, Susan Meyer and Karen Sauvigné . . . brainstormed to invent a name for their newly identified issue: 'sexual harassment.' " In Susan Brownmiller and Dolores Alexander, "From Carmita Wood to Anita Hill," *Ms.* magazine, vol. 2, no. 4 (January–February 1992), pp. 70–71.

P. 9 "The earliest media use . . .": Enid Nemy, "Women Begin to Speak Out Against Sexual Harassment at Work," *New York Times*, Aug. 19, 1975, p. 38.

P. 9 "Eleanor Holmes Norton . . .": Norton, currently a professor of law at Georgetown University and the nonvoting delegate to Congress for the District of Columbia, is a pioneering civil rights attorney and co-founder of the National Black Feminist Organization.

P. 9 "Unwelcome sexual advances . . .": Equal Employment Opportunity Commission (EEOC), 1980: Guidelines on Discrimination Because of Sex. 29 C.F.R.1604.

P. 10 "the following seven forms . . .": U.S. Merit Systems Protection Board, *Sexual Harassment of Federal Workers: An Update* (Washington, DC: U.S. Government Printing Office, 1988), chap. 2. (This document is available on the Internet. See this book's World Wide Web site for the link.) Although the Merit Systems study's categories have been widely adopted, other classifications are being developed as researchers refine behavioral categories in order to ascertain the true extent and impact of harassment. For instance, James Gruber has developed a typology of eleven forms of behavior within three main categories—Verbal Requests, Verbal Comments, and Nonverbal Displays— each of which can range from more to less severe. See James E. Gruber, "A Typology of Personal and Environmental Sexual Harassment: Research and

Policy Implications for the 1990s," *Sex Roles: A Journal of Research*, vol. 26, no. 11–12 (June 1992), p. 447. Louise F. Fitzgerald and Alayne J. Ormerod classify harassment as Gender Harassment, Seductive Behavior, Sexual Bribery, Sexual Coercion, and Sexual Assault or Rape. See Louise F. Fitzgerald and Alayne J. Ormerod, "Perceptions of Sexual Harassment: The Influence of Gender and Academic Context," *Psychology of Women Quarterly*, vol. 15, no. 2 (June 1991), p. 281.

P. 11 "That's what you've got to expect . . .": Quoted in Jean Zimmerman, *Tailspin: Women at War in the Wake of Tailhook* (New York: Doubleday, 1995), p. 27.

P. 11 "nearly equal numbers of Republicans and Democrats . . .": An interesting account of the congressional politics and voting involved in passing the 1964 Civil Rights Act can be found in Jo Freeman, "How 'Sex' Got Into Title VII: Persistent Opportunism as a Maker of Public Policy," *Law and Inequality: A Journal of Theory and Practice*, vol. 9 (1991), pp. 163–84. (This article is available on the Internet; see this book's World Wide Web site for the link.)

P. 11 "race, color, religion, sex . . .": Title VII of the 1964 U.S. Civil Rights Act can be found in 42 U.S.C. §2000e.

P. 11 "it was not until 1976 . . .": *Williams v. Saxbe*, 413 F.Supp. 654 (D.D.C. 1976). For some of the legal scholarship that helped establish sexual harassment as a form of sex discrimination, see Catharine A. MacKinnon, *Sexual Harassment of Working Women: A Case of Sex Discrimination* (New Haven: Yale University Press, 1979). Also: J. Ralph Lindgren and Nadine Taub, *The Law of Sex Discrimination*, 2d ed. Minneapolis/St. Paul: West Publishing Co., 1993.

P. 12 "to be decided by the U.S. Supreme Court . . .": *Meritor v. Vinson*, 477 U.S. 57 (1986).

P. 12 "revisited the hostile environment concept . . .": *Harris v. Forklift Systems*, 114 S.Ct.367 (1993). The full text of Justice O'Connor's opinion, as well as concurring opinions filed by Justices Ruth Bader Ginsburg and Antonin Scalia, can be found in Appendix D. (All recent Supreme Court opinions can also be found on the Internet; see this book's World Wide Web site for the link.)

P. 18 "the judge accepted the normalcy . . .": *Corne v. Bausch & Lomb*, 390 F.Supp. 161 (D. Ariz. 1975).

P. 18 "as Lieutenant Coughlin's admiral put it . . .": Zimmerman, *Tailspin*, p. 19.

P. 23 "*sex-role spillover* . . ." Barbara A. Gutek and Aaron G. Cohen, "Sex Ratios, Sex Role Spillover, and Sex at Work: A Comparison of Men's and Women's Experiences," *Human Relations*, vol. 40 (1987), pp. 97–115.

## Chapter 3: Sexual Boundaries: Masculine and Feminine

P. 30 "about the relational needs . . .": See Deborah Tannen, *You Just Don't Understand: Women and Men in Conversation* (New York: Ballantine, 1991); Carol Gilligan, *In a Different Voice: Psychological Theory and Women's Development* (Cambridge:

Harvard University Press, 1982); Lyn Mikel Brown and Carol Gilligan, *Meeting at the Crossroads: Women's Psychology and Girls' Development* (New York: Ballantine, 1993); and Peggy Orenstein, *School Girls: Young Women, Self-Esteem, and the Confidence Gap* (New York: Doubleday, 1994).

P. 31 "Recent research on sexual fantasies . . .": See Bruce J. Ellis and Donald Symons, "Sex Differences in Sexual Fantasy: An Evolutionary Psychological Approach," *Journal of Sex Research*, vol. 27 (1990), pp. 527–55.

P. 31 "capacities that the culture considers masculine . . .": A good introduction to C. G. Jung's concepts can be found in his autobiography, *Memories, Dreams, Reflections* (New York: Vintage Books, 1989). Jung discusses the animus and anima more extensively in *Two Essays on Analytical Psychology*, 2d ed. (Princeton: Princeton University Press, 1966). For a contemporary treatment of Jungian concepts, including anima and animus, that includes modern thinking about gender roles, see Andrew Samuels, *Jung and the Post-Jungians* (New York: Routledge, 1985).

P. 33 "I cried over you last night . . .": *Ellison v. Brady*, p. 207 of this book.

P. 41 "the underlying threat of violence . . .": *Ellison v. Brady*, p. 214 of this book.

P. 49 "Conduct considered harmless by many today . . .": *Ellison v. Brady*, p. 215n of this book.

## Chapter 4: Sexual Fantasies: How Inner Life Affects Outer Boundaries

P. 55 "some of the more common forms of sexual harassment . . .": U.S. Merit Systems Protection Board, *Sexual Harassment.*

P. 56 "I have enjoyed you . . ." *Ellison v. Brady*, p. 208 of this book.

P. 58 "the animus is a way of identifying strengths . . .": For a distinctly feminine Jungian view of the animus, see M. Esther Harding, *The Way of All Women* (New York: Putnam, 1971). An excellent contemporary Freudian view of feminine psychology can be found in Charlotte Krause Prozan, *Feminist Psychoanalytic Psychotherapy* (Northvale, NJ: Jason Aronson, 1992).

## Chapter 5: How Harassment Happens: Sexual Coercion, Varieties of Boundary Crossings, and Gender Harassment

P. 73 "Vinson's supervisor made repeated demands . . .": Quoted in *Ellison v. Brady*, p. 209 of this book.

P. 74 "Paula Coughlin's multimillion-dollar jury verdict . . .": Benjamin A. Holden, "Hilton Hotels Loses $5 Million Verdict in Tailhook Case," *Wall Street Journal*, Nov. 1, 1994.

P. 75 "A unanimous Supreme Court in 1993 . . .": *Harris v. Forklift Systems*, 114 U.S. 367 (1993), see Appendix D of this book.

P. 76 "A woman who worked at a video store . . .": From Melissa Monson, "Defining the Situation: Sexual Harassment or Everyday Rudeness?" Paper presented at the Conference of the Sociologists Against Sexual Harassment, 1994.

P. 82 "he gave Ellison a tour of his house . . ." *Ellison v. Brady*, p. 207 of this book.

P. 84 "the Senate Ethics Committee resolution for the investigation of Senator Packwood . . .": Helen Dewar, "Panel Details Packwood Allegations," *Washington Post*, May 18, 1995.

P. 87 "gender harassment is a workplace spillover . . .": For a thorough discussion of gender harassment as a form of violence against women, see Fitzgerald's chapters on violence at work in Mary P. Koss et al., *No Safe Haven: Male Violence Against Women at Home, at Work, and in the Community* (Washington, DC: American Psychological Association, 1994). For an excellent cultural history of violence against women, see Pamela Cooper-White, *The Cry of Tamar: Violence Against Women and the Church's Response* (Minneapolis: Fortress Press, 1995).

## Chapter 6: A Guide for Men: Preventing Sexual Harassment and Responding to a Complaint

P. 100 "only 5 percent of cases . . .": U.S. Merit Systems Protection Board, *Sexual Harassment*, chap. 3.

P. 101 "procedures for investigating it . . .": For an excellent outline of investigation procedures, see Susan G. Kemp, Richard J. Curiale, and Stephen J. Hirschfeld, *Stopping Sexual Harassment: An Employer's Guide* (Sacramento: California Chamber of Commerce, 1993), pp. 90–121.

P. 105 "men are much less likely to experience it . . .": See Barbara A. Gutek, "Responses to Sexual Harassment," in Stuart Oskamp and Mark Costanzo, eds., *Gender Issues in Contemporary Society* (Newbury Park, CA: Sage Publications, 1993), p. 203.

## Chapter 7: A Guide for Women: Taking Charge of Boundaries and Initiating a Complaint

P. 110 "deferential and pleasant . . .": See Deborah Tannen, *Talking from 9 to 5* (New York: William Morrow, 1994), especially chap. 8, for an application to the workplace of men's and women's different communicational styles spelled out in *You Just Don't Understand*. Also, see Denise Lach and Patricia A. Gwartney-Gibbs, "Sociological Perspectives on Sexual Harassment and Workplace Dispute Resolution," *Journal of Vocational Behavior* (Special Issue: Sexual Harassment in the Workplace), vol. 42 (1993), pp. 102–15.

P. 116 "the Chevron Corporation agreed to settle . . .": Tamar Lewin, "Chevron

Agrees to Pay $2.2 Million in Settlement of Sexual Harassment Case," *New York Times,* Feb. 22, 1995.

P. 121 "effects of childhood trauma." See Judith Lewis Herman, *Trauma and Recovery* (New York: Basic Books, 1992), for a masterful account of this subject.

P. 121 "a positive feminine role model . . .": For an intimate portrait of the psychotherapy process between two women, see Virginia Beane Rutter, *Woman Changing Woman: Feminine Psychology Re-conceived Through Myth and Experience* (San Francisco: HarperSanFrancisco, 1993).

P. 126 "a prelude to violent sexual assault . . ." *Ellison v. Brady,* p. 214 of this book.

P. 127 "approximately 90 percent of perceived episodes . . .": U.S. Merit Systems Protection Board, *Sexual Harassment of Federal Workers: An Update,* chap. 3.

P. 127 "Diffidence about confronting can also . . .": See Stephanie Riger, "Gender Dilemmas in Sexual Harassment: Policies and Procedures," in Sherri Marie Matteo, ed., *American Women in the Nineties: Today's Critical Issues* (Boston: Northeastern University Press, 1993), pp. 213–34. See also Lach and Gwartney-Gibbs, "Sociological Perspectives."

P. 129 "Educational institutions that receive . . .": For an overview of Title IX sexual harassment, see American Association of University Women, *Hostile Hallways: The AAUW Survey on Sexual Harassment in America's Schools* (Washington, DC: AAUW Educational Foundation, 1993).

P. 135 "Sexual harassment lawsuits . . .": A wealth of practical information about pursuing EEOC and other legal options can be found in William Petrocelli and Barbara Kate Repa, *Sexual Harassment on the Job: What It Is and How to Stop It,* 2d ed. (Berkeley: Nolo Press, 1994).

## Chapter 8: A Guide for Organizations: Humanizing the Workplace

P. 140 "twenty-three articles about sexual harassment indexed for 1994 . . .": PsycInfo and ABI/Inform are available on many university-based computer networks, as well as through commercial on-line service providers.

P. 142 "a new 'local social norm' . . .": Global social norms and local social norms are related to sexual harassment issues in John B. Pryor, Christine M. LaVite, and Lynnette M. Stoller, "A Social Psychological Analysis of Sexual Harassment: The Person/Situation Interaction," *Journal of Vocational Behavior* (Special Issue: Sexual Harassment in the Workplace), vol. 42 (1993), pp. 68–83.

P. 142 "When Judge Beezer writes . . .": *Ellison v. Brady,* p. 215 of this book.

## Chapter 10: Boundaries Everywhere

P. 169 "peer sexual harassment complaints . . .": Julie Gannon Shoop, "Beyond Horseplay: Students Sue Schools Over Sexual Harassment," *Trial*, vol. 30 (1994), pp. 12–14.

P. 169 "Programs like these . . .": See Nan D. Stein and Lisa Sjostrom, *Flirting or Hurting: A Teacher's Guide on Student-to-Student Sexual Harassment in Schools* (Washington, DC: National Education Association, 1994).

P. 170 "early adolescence is a crucial time . . .": See note to Chapter 3, p. 30. See also Carol Gilligan, Annie G. Rogers, and Deborah L. Tolman, eds., *Women, Girls and Psychotherapy: Reframing Resistance* (New York: Haworth Press, 1991). Also see Mary Pipher, *Reviving Ophelia: Saving the Selves of Adolescent Girls* (New York: Ballantine, 1994).

P. 172 "sexual harassment or Title IX officers, student advocates . . .": For a first hand view of the complexities of this role, see Susan Hippensteele, "Advocacy and Student Victims of Sexual Harassment," in B. Sandler and R. Shoop, eds., *Sexual Harassment on Campus: A Guide for Administrators, Faculty, and Students* (Boston: Allyn and Bacon, 1996).

P. 173 "sex between a student and . . .": See Peter Rutter, *Sex in the Forbidden Zone: When Men in Power—Therapists, Doctors, Clergy, Teachers, and Others—Betray Women's Trust* (New York: Fawcett Crest, 1991).

P. 176 "date or acquaintance rape . . .": See Jean O'Gorman Hughes and Bernice R. Sandler, *"Friends" Raping Friends: Could It Happen to You?* (Washington, DC: Project on the Status and Education of Women, Association of American Colleges, 1987).

# INDEX

# ABOUT THE AUTHOR

Peter Rutter, M.D., is a board-certified psychiatrist, an associate clinical professor of psychiatry at the University of California Medical School, San Francisco, and a former chair of the ethics committee of the C. G. Jung Institute of San Francisco. He received a Distinguished Teacher Award in Health and Medical Sciences from the University of California, Berkeley, has published articles and chapters in professional journals and books, and is the author of the book *Sex in the Forbidden Zone*. Dr. Rutter is in clinical practice, and teaches and consults internationally in the areas of sexual harassment, sexual exploitation of professional trust relationships, and ethical standards and procedures.